ENVIRONMENTAL POISONS IN OUR FOOD

ENVIRONMENTAL POISONS IN OUR FOOD

J. GORDON MILLICHAP, M.D., F.R.C.P.

Professor Emeritus of Pediatrics and Neurology,
Northwestern University Medical School,
Children's Memorial Hospital,
Chicago, Illinois

Formerly, Consultant in Pediatric Neurology,
Mayo Clinic, Rochester, Minnesota

P N B • PUBLISHER
Chicago • London

Published and Distributed Throughout the World by

PNB • Publishers
P.O. Box 11391
Chicago, Illinois 60611, U.S.A.

Printed in the U.S.A.

ISBN 0-9629115-7-7
Library of Congress Catalog Card Number: 92-91280

Affectionately inscribed to my dear wife,
Nancy,
and to our four fine sons,
Martin, Paul, Gordon, and John.

PREFACE

Fourteen million or more children less than seven years of age are exposed to lead in the environment in the United States. Seventeen percent have blood lead levels sufficient to cause serious deficits in intelligence and disorders of behavior that persist through adolescence to adulthood.

Lead is just one of many poisons that contaminate our food and water and pose potential risks to the health of both children and adult populations. Despite governmental regulations designed to control hazardous wastes and the use of poisonous pesticides and insecticides in agriculture, dangerous levels of mercury, PCB, DDT, and other toxic residues continue to contaminate our inland lakes and waterways. Lake fish, especially large trout and salmon, are considered unsafe to eat in Illinois, Wisconsin, Indiana, and Michigan. For a fisherman to eat his catch, he risks damage to his nervous system from mercury and the development of cancer from industrial residues.

Statistics from the American Cancer Society show that one in three, or 83 million Americans, living in 1992 will develop cancer in their life spans.

The expected number of new cases of liver and stomach cancer, the types most likely to be related to food and water toxicants, is 40,000 in 1992. In the past 60 years, deaths from cancer have increased from 143/100,000 to 170/100,000 population annually. Dietary factors and pesticide residues may be responsible for 30 percent of reported human cancers or even as many as 60 percent in men.

The commercial processing of food is a major source of contamination, with additives, PBBs, and bacterial toxins. The use of cobalt chloride as a foam stabilizer in the manufacture of beer in the 1960s had tragic consequences. More recently, a major distributor recalled cases of their bottled water that had been tainted with benzene used in cleaning tanks. Even the plastic food packaging materials have potential carcinogenic properties and require regulatory controls. Apart from the Chernobyl disaster and similar nuclear risks, we are now asked to accept the "benefits" of food irradiation in the processing of our food.

As consumers, we have little or no control over potential food risks introduced via the environment, methods of agriculture, commercial processing, in restaurants, or from packaging materials. However , we can limit the risks of food poisoning by care in the preparation and storage of food in the kitchen, the avoidance of an overzealous intake of certain vitamins and minerals, and an understanding of the hazards of food allergies for those individuals with asthma and sensitivity reactions.

A recent physician sponsored survey showed that scientific information on mercury, PCB and other food toxins was not readily available to practicing family doctors. Neither the physicians interviewed nor their patients fully appreciated the health risks of environmental pollutants. A comprehensive yet practical account of the subject of environmental food poisons was urgently needed.

This book is written for the consumer and for interested members of the medical and public health professions. It provides an awareness and a better understanding of the potential health risks from environmental toxins in our food and water, the symptoms and signs of illnesses caused by them, and ways to avoid their harmful effects. The subject matter covered in fourteen chapters includes food poisoning with lead and trace metals, pesticide and insecticide residues, foodborne and waterborne infections and toxins, food additives, excess vitamin toxicity, alcoholic and caffeine beverages, and food allergies. Suggestions are provided to help reduce the risks of food poisoning at the consumer level.

The regulation of our food and water supplies and improvements in the safety of our environment are the responsibility and essential role of good government. We can anticipate programs to achieve this goal in this decade.

J. Gordon Millichap, M.D., F.R.C.P.

ACKNOWLEDGMENTS

In addition to material based on the author's medical practice and research, various sources of information are cited in the references. In particular, I wish to acknowledge the valuable material made available through the library of the Northwestern University Medical School and derived from the following publications: Nutritional Toxicology, Vols I, II, and III, Academic Press: the National Research Council; the World Health Organization; the Environmental Protection Agency; Food Additives Handbook and Bibliography, Van Nostrand and Orynx Press; Cecil Textbook of Medicine, WB Saunders; Nelson Textbook of Pediatrics, WB Saunders; Mandell et al Principles and Practice of Infectious Diseases, Churchill Livingston; and the Pharmacological Basis of Therapeutics by my mentors, Louis S Goodman and the late Alfred Gilman, and published by Macmillan.

I also wish to thank my wife, Nancy Millichap, who proofread the manuscript and offered constructive suggestions; my son, John, who facilitated my introduction to the word processor; and my son, Gordon, who applied his artistic talents to the cover design and helped choose the "Sunfish" picture, courtesy of Hunting and Fishing Library, Minnetonka, MN.

J. Gordon Millichap, M.D., F.R.C.P.

TABLE OF CONTENTS

ENVIRONMENTAL POISONS IN OUR FOOD

CHAPTER 1

LEAD POISONING

"Pica, an abnormal craving for unnatural items of food, is a prelude to plumbism."
J.G.Millichap et al. Lancet 2:360, 1952.

Increased lead absorption and lead poisoning (plumbism) affect all ages, but children are most susceptible and may be exposed even during fetal life and infancy. The recognition of potential sources of lead contamination of food and water in the environment should lead to the prevention or reduction of morbidity and mortality from this dangerous and hidden hazard. There is no biological function or need for lead in our food or bodies, and there is no such thing as a "normal" lead level in the blood.

Lead is a toxic substance that damages the nervous system, the blood, the kidneys, and other organs. In view of new scientific data that has uncovered subtle and sustained long-term effects of lead on cognition, school performance, and behavior of children, pediatricians and public health officials have responded with a renewed and vigorous effort to diagnose cases of lead poisoning early and to eliminate lead from the environment of children and pregnant mothers. The goal is the prevention of this ***silent epidemic.***

SOURCES OF LEAD

The sources of lead intoxication are different in children and adults and even in infants, toddlers, and older children.

Infants may be exposed to lead in formula prepared with lead-contaminated water, especially if the water is "soft" and is obtained from a lead-lined hot water cistern.

Toddlers are prone to "pica", a craving for unnatural items of food, and the ingestion of paint chips is the most common source of lead poisoning in children aged 18 through 30 months. Children with a tendency to pica are especially at risk. Multilayered chips of old lead pigment paints may contain 20,000-100,000 mcg Pb/cm^2. House dust in old houses may average from 600-3,000 mcg Pb/g, and garden soil can contain 2,000-16,000 mcg Pb/g. These are the major sources of exposure to lead in young children in the United States, and the hand-to-mouth activity common to toddlers is a predisposing factor in this age group.

Older Children and Adolescents are poisoned by the sniffing of leaded gasoline for hedonistic purposes. They may also be exposed to fumes from burning painted wood or casings of storage batteries used for heating living quarters in socioeconomically deprived areas of cities. Aerosol exposure is especially hazardous, since approximately 40 per cent of inhaled lead is absorbed. Organic tetraethyl lead in gasoline has a proclivity for the nervous system, causing an acute lead encephalopathy manifested by coma and convulsions.

An unusual source of ingested lead in children is making spitballs from newspaper. Newspapers contain up to 4000 ppm lead and can contribute significant amounts of lead to children with this habit.

Adults have occupational sources of lead exposure as seen in metal smelter workers or miners, welders, storage battery workers, pottery makers, ship builders, auto workers, paint manufacturers, house painters and renovators, and those employed in printing industries. Demolition workers and employees in firing ranges have been poisoned from excessive aerosol exposure to lead containing dusts. It has been estimated that about one million American workers are exposed to abnormal quantities of lead in their occupational environments.

Pottery with lead glaze and kettles and cans with lead-soldered joints release lead into food and water when acidic fluids such as fruit preserves and juices are stored or cooked in them. Old pottery mugs and antique kettles are ornamental in the kitchen but should be left on the shelf.

With the increase in crime and gun shot wounds, bullets retained in tissues and particularly in joints or bone are a significant source of lead poisoning. The interval between the penetration and lodging of the bullet and clinical signs of lead poisoning may range from 2 days to 40 years. Synovial fluid in joints is an excellent solvent for lead and facilitates the diffusion of lead into the blood stream and other organ systems.

Sporadic cases of plumbism have been traced to other sources of high concentrations of lead, including lead shot from hunted fowl or rabbit, the inadvertent swallowing of fishing or curtain weights and heads of lead soldiers or other lead toys, and the ingestion of lead contaminated folk and herbal medicines, aphrodisiacs, and Asiatic cosmetics. In the southern United States where whiskey is made in stills and condensers containing lead, up to 90 per cent of this moonshine is potentially toxic and is a source of lead poisoning.

Before the Industrial Revolution the total body content of lead was about 2 mg; in industrialized societies today this figure has increased 100 times. Of 200 mcg of lead ingested each day, about 5 to 10 per cent is absorbed, and the amounts are even higher in children. In malnourished children with deficiencies of iron, calcium, magnesium, and zinc, the absorption and potential for toxicity from lead exposure are increased. Diets suboptimal in iron and calcium are prevalent among children in low income groups.

LEAD CONTENT OF FOODS

Determinations of food items sampled from various markets in the United States showed that canned tomatoes had the highest mean lead content, followed by canned beans with tomato sauce, peas, and peaches in decreasing order. Sugar, raw potatoes, margarine, and white flour had the lowest mean values of lead. The raw agricultural commodities with the highest residues of lead were corn, wheat, soybeans, and tomatoes.

The estimated daily intake of lead from food for adult Americans is about 250 mcg (Bureau of Foods, 1975). This estimate is below the values of 500-600 mcg set as amounts that would cause concern. In another study based on food consumption patterns, fruits and vegetables constitute 78 per cent of the total lead intake.

A survey of baby foods made by the Bureau of Foods, 1975, revealed that orange juice had the highest mean lead content (380 ppb), followed by apple juice (320 ppb), applesauce (160 ppb), and peaches (94 ppb) in decreasing order. Vegetables and beef (70 ppb) and mixed vegetables (72 ppb) had the lowest lead contents. The estimated dietary intake of lead for selected age groups of infants and toddlers was 80 mcg for 2 month-old infants, 63 mcg for 6 month, 100 mcg for 1 year, and 115 mcg for 2-year-old children.

Lead residues in food are influenced by several factors:

•Biological uptake of lead from soils into plants eaten by animals and man.

•Lead arsenate pesticides used in horticulture.

•Food processing and storage in cans. Lead contents correlated with the seam length/volume ratio of cans of viscous tomato paste. When stored open for 24 hours, the lead content of samples closest to the seam was 10-fold higher than the content of samples taken farthest from the seam.

•Location where vegetables are grown in relation to major highways. An inverse relationship between distance from the road and lead content has been observed. Samples taken near the Eisenhower Expressway in Chicago contained 685 ppm of lead, of which 50 per cent could be washed off.

LEAD IN DRINKING WATER

Lead in drinking water contributes between 10 and 20 percent of total lead exposure in young children. Water as a source of lead poisoning may increase in relative importance as abatement programs reduce exposure from lead-based paint and urban soil and dust. (See Chapter 9 on Waterborne Diseases for further details).

The U.S. Environmental Protection Agency (EPA) estimated in 1986 that some 40 million Americans were drinking water that contained potentially hazardous levels of lead. Until this year, the EPA limit for lead levels in drinking water was 50 ppb. The new limit has been set at 15 ppb. Recent tests of water from household taps in Illinois failed to meet the new Federal standards in a number of townships. Adding phosphate to the main water supply to control corrosion of plumbing is one solution to the problem. The replacement of lead service pipes would be a more costly alternative.

A 1986 law banned the use of leaded solder on pipes that carry drinking water. Much of household plumbing consists of copper pipes connected by lead-containing solder. The newer the plumbing installation, the greater the risk of lead leaching from the pipes. Older pipes have developed a protective coating of deposits. Brass faucets are an additional source of lead, particularly if the water is soft and more corrosive.

ROLE OF NUTRITIONAL FACTORS

Many nutritional factors can affect the absorption of lead in the diet. Deficiencies of protein, calcium, phosphorus, vitamin E, iron, zinc, and selenium can increase the severity of lead toxicity, whereas a high protein diet, and ascorbic acid and iron supplements have a protective effect. Caution must be used in prescribing health food supplements of calcium and other minerals, since some prepared from bones of old horses have been contaminated with lead.

The quantity and type of dietary fat may be important in lead intoxication. Butterfat causes an increase in lead absorption, whereas fats containing polyunsaturated fatty acids (sunflower oil) have little effect. Lecithin, bile salts, and choline may stimulate the uptake of lead by the intestine. Milk in the diet influences susceptibility to lead poisoning by providing calcium and phosphorus, and generous portions of carrots and cabbage are reported to increase lead excretion in the urine.

Of all these dietary factors listed, iron deficiency is probably the most important nutritional problem that predisposes young children to lead toxicity.

INCIDENCE AND EPIDEMIOLOGY

Seventeen per cent of children in the United States aged 6 months to 6 years are reported to have blood lead levels greater than 10 to15 mcg/dL. The Agency for Toxic Substances and Disease Registry (ATSDR) has defined the threshold for neurobehavioral toxicity for lead as 10 mcg/dL. As sustained lead levels rise above this threshold, children exposed are at a progressively increasing risk for future cognitive and behavioral abnormalities which can lead to school problems and learning deficits.

Chronic lead absorption is most prevalent in pre-school children living in old, deteriorated housing. According to the ATSDR, the number of potentially exposed children younger than 7 years of age living in old housing with lead paint is about 12 million. The US Census Bureau recorded 42 million dwelling units built before 1950 and still occupied in 1983. Lead-containing paint and the highest levels of lead in surface soil and interior household dust are found in and around this type of housing. Exposure to house dust containing greater than 1,000 mcg Pb/g of dust in a pre-school child with hand-to-mouth activity can produce blood lead levels in the toxic range of 16-60 mcg/dL. More severe degrees of poisoning are associated with pica and repeated ingestion of lead paint chips or some uncommon inhaled source of lead.

SYMPTOMS AND SIGNS

The developing nervous system is most sensitive to the toxic effects of lead in the fetus and young child. Lead crosses the placenta and is responsible for spontaneous abortion and miscarriage. It also causes stunting of fetal growth and childhood stature by effects on growth hormone secretion. Lead exposure may result in chromosome anomalies and reduced sperm counts. The principal toxic effects of lead occur in the nervous system, the blood, kidney, and gastrointestinal tract.

Nervous System. Central nervous system symptoms and signs are vague at first and include irritability, incoordination, memory lapses, sleep disturbances, listlessness, headache, and dizziness. Symptoms of brain damage may occur with blood levels of 25 to 60 mcg Pb/dL or less in children.

The long-term effects of low dose lead exposure (10 to 25 mcg/dL blood lead levels) during early childhood have been correlated with impairment of academic success at a later age. Studies have shown a failure to graduate from high school, lower class standing, absenteeism, and dyslexia in adolescents exposed to lead at an early age. Deficits in vocabulary, fine motor skills, coordination, and reaction time have been reported.

The lead content of dentin in teeth shed at ages 6 and 7 years showed a positive correlation with neuro-behavioral impairments as measured in young adulthood. Young people with dentin lead levels greater than 20 ppm (parts per million) had a markedly higher risk of dropping out of high school and of having a reading disability as compared with those with dentin lead levels less than 10 ppm. Exposure to lead even in children who remain asymptomatic may have an important and enduring effect on brain functioning and learning.

More serious and striking manifestations of lead poisoning include syncope or fainting attacks, disorientation, mental impairment, schizophrenic-like psychosis, ataxia, vomiting, severe headache, seizures, blindness, and coma. *Acute encephalopathy* is more common in children than in adults and carries a poor prognosis. The mortality rate is high and brain damage is frequent, with persistent neurologic sequelae including seizures, paralyses, and mental retardation.

The spinal cord is affected rarely, producing a syndrome that resembles amyotrophic lateral sclerosis (Lou Gehrig's disease). Some studies have shown that patients with Lou Gehrig's disease report exposure to lead and mercury, the consumption of large amounts of milk, and participation in athletics and manual labor, factors that may increase susceptibility to lead-induced paralyses.

The peripheral nervous system is involved more often in adults than children and paralyses of the muscles supplied by the radial nerve result in weakness of finger extension and wrist drop. In adults leg paralyses are exceptional, but the converse is true in children who may present with weakness and wasting of the muscles of the feet or sometimes of the quadriceps.

Abdominal Symptoms. Intermittent abdominal cramps or colic are associated with nausea, vomiting, loss of appetite, and constipation. The pain may simulate appendicitis and other surgical intestinal disorders that must be considered in diagnosis.

Other symptoms include anemia, kidney failure, and joint pains. A blue line on the gums is found in 20 per cent of adults with chronic lead exposure but is infrequent in children.

DIAGNOSIS OF LEAD POISONING

Symptoms are nonspecific and mimic other diseases. A high index of suspicion is important in making the diagnosis. Plumbism should be suspected in a child with pica, living in an old, deteriorated house, who presents with abdominal pain, vomiting, irritability, seizures, or anemia. The environment should be examined for sources of lead and early diagnosis depends on laboratory tests which supplement the clinical acumen of the physician.

The blood lead level is the screening test of choice. An acceptable blood lead is less than 10 mcg Pb/dL, and risks of toxicity and neurological residua increase in stages according to lead levels: Stage I, 10-20 mcg/dL; stage II, 20-45 mcg/dL; stage III, 40-70 mcg/dL; and stage IV, more than 70 mcg/dL. Patients show a varying susceptibility to lead and become symptomatic at different levels. A high lead screening test is not pathognomonic of lead encephalopathy in a comatose child, and alternative diagnoses such as cerebral tumor and viral encephalitis must be considered before specific treatment is initiated.

Erythrocyte protoporphyrin (EP) determinations are not sufficiently reliable as a screening test, and will not identify children with the lower elevations of blood lead between 10 and 25 mcg/dL. Abnormally high levels of EP are found in iron deficiency anemia, with or without lead poisoning, and the test is not specific. EP levels are obtained before chelation therapy and are used concurrently with blood lead levels in following the course and response to treatment.

An *X-ray of the abdomen* may reveal radiopaque flecks of lead from recently ingested paint, and an *X-ray of the long bones* such as femur or tibia will have bands of increased density or "lead lines" in children chronically exposed but not in patients with acute encephalopathy. These roentgenograms , tests of hair and fingernails for lead, and examination of red blood cells for basophilic stippling are of secondary importance to the blood lead level in diagnosis and are not included in the routine workup of a patient with suspected lead poisoning.

The CaNaEDTA Mobilization Test is used to determine whether a child diagnosed with lead poisoning and with a blood lead level of 25-44 mcg/dL will respond to chelation therapy with a brisk lead excretion in the urine. This test is not indicated in children with a blood lead of 45 mcg/dL or greater, which requires immediate chelation to avoid potential neurologic sequelae.

TREATMENT OF LEAD POISONING

The removal of the child from the source of lead and removal of the lead hazard from the environment are the cornerstones of therapy. Pregnant women should also evacuate the premises until the abatement of the lead paint has been completed. The removal of the hazard is usually the responsibility of the local health agency and the landlord and should be performed by professionals.

Lead Abatement. The Environmental Protection Agency (EPA) recently launched a series of training and certification programs around the country to teach abatement skills to contractors. Employees should wear protective gear and vacuuming should be performed with a high-efficiency particle accumulator. The average cost of home lead abatement is $7,000 and a national cleanup program could cost an estimated $100 billion.

Lead laws and abatement regulations in some states are very stringent, leading to costly and trying circumstances for property owners and realtors. Laws address disclosure of lead hazards in properties for sale, and contracts are required to warn buyers that older houses may contain lead and recommend that buyers opt for a lead inspection before the purchase.

When a lead paint source of exposure is discovered, the premises should be professionally vacuumed, scrubbed with high-phosphate detergents, and then repainted with unleaded paint. Play in dirt adjacent to the housing should be avoided. The patient is tested periodically to determine progress of lead levels, and other children in the household are also examined for evidence of plumbism.

Treatment Regimens. Most children detected with increased blood lead levels are asymptomatic and fit the classifications of stages I, II, or III lead absorption or intoxication. For those in stages I and II, an improved diet including iron to treat anemia may be sufficient. Patients in stages III and IV require chelation therapy, including those who are asymptomatic.

Chelation therapy . The chelating agents used in treating children with lead poisoning are shown in the Table 1-1.

TABLE 1-1. Chelating Therapies for Lead Poisoning.

Product Name	***Generic Name***	***Abbreviation***
CaNa Versenate	Edetate di-NaCa	CaNaEDTA
BAL in Oil	Dimercaprol	BAL
Chemet	Succimer	DMSA

CaNaEDTA is employed in patients with blood lead levels above 45 mcg/dL and in those with acute encephalopathy. It is administered for 5 days, preferably by continuous intravenous infusion. BAL is used to initiate chelation therapy in patients with more severe intoxication and with blood lead levels above 70 mcg/dL. Therapy with BAL is supplemented with CaNaEDTA.

Succimer (DMSA) is preferred for patients with milder intoxications and blood lead levels above 45 and below 70 mcg/dL. It is not FDA approved for the prophylaxis of lead poisoning in areas of high risk exposure or for treatment of patients who are symptomatic or have blood lead levels of 70 mcg/dL or higher. It is administered orally and allows the option of outpatient management and lower health care costs. Succimer chelates are excreted in the urine, and adequate hydration is essential to maintain good urine flow. The drug has a "rotten egg" sulfur odor which is a disadvantage. Unlike CaEDTA, DMSA does not induce acute zinc depletion, and it is more effective than CaEDTA in lowering lead content of brain, kidney, and blood.

Electrolyte solutions are administered intravenously to correct losses due to vomiting and dehydration, *mannitol* may be required to reduce intracranial pressure, and *diazepam* is used to control acute prolonged seizures in patients with acute encephalopathy.

Effective long term management of lead poisoning derived from paint requires the cooperative efforts of health department personnel, social worker, psychologist , and pediatrician or family practitioner. Pica and hand-to-mouth activity that predispose to plumbism may be benefited by behavior modification.

PROGNOSIS

Even relatively low lead levels greater than 10 to 15 mcg/dL, if sustained during early childhood, may result in subtle injury to the nervous system that is manifested as learning and behavioral problems in later childhood and young adults. Sequelae are related to the degree and duration of excessive lead ingestion and absorption. Survivors of acute encephalopathy may be mentally retarded, and suffer from seizures and paralyses. Prevention or early diagnosis and effective therapeutic measures are essential for improvements in the prognosis of this common environmental hazard.

PREVENTION

Public Health Agencies in the United States have attempted to reduce the risks of lead exposure and poisoning by enforcing drinking water standards for lead, reducing the lead content of canned foods, and in 1988, eliminating lead additives in gasoline. The lead in residential paints was banned by the United States Consumer Product Safety Commission in 1977, but lead-based paint and lead-contaminated dusts remain the primary sources of lead exposure for children.

Lead remains in approximately 74 per cent of all private dwellings built before 1978, and housing built before 1950 is at even greater risk of having interior lead-based paint. Methods of prevention of lead ingestion or inhalation from these and other sources include the following:

•Children and pregnant women should not be allowed to remain in an old house that is undergoing renovation or removal of paint.

•If lead in plumbing is suspected, water from a hot water tap should not be used for drinking or food preparation. The cold water tap should be flushed for several minutes each morning or until there is a noticeable change in the temperature of the water before any is consumed.

•Infant formula should not be mixed with water from the hot tap.

• Outside play areas should be located away from houses and buildings and highways with heavy traffic, so that concentrations of lead paint dust and leaded gasoline spills in soil are minimized.

•Food grown in city gardens should be meticulously washed to remove contaminating lead dust and soil.

•Food from opened cans should be transferred immediately into glass or plastic containers for storage in the refrigerator.

•Bread wrappers are printed with lead based paint and should not be turned inside out and reused.

Screening. In many States, physicians or health care providers are required by law to screen children 6 months to 6 years of age for lead poisoning, in accordance with guidelines and criteria set forth by the American Academy of Pediatrics.

The Center for Disease Control (CDC) guidelines (Oct 7, 1991) changed the definition of lead poisoning to a blood lead level greater than or equal to 10 mcg/dL. Because the Erythrocyte Protoporphyrin level is not adequately sensitive to identify children with elevated blood lead levels below 25 mcg/dL, the screening test of choice is a blood lead measurement. Capillary blood specimens are more practical than venous samples for screening purposes but they may be contaminated by lead dust on the child's hand. Diagnostic blood levels must be measured on venous samples.

All children are at risk for lead poisoning in our industrialized society and it is recommended that all children be screened. Those children ages 6 months to 6 years and those living in older housing are the highest priority for screening. Assessment of the risk of lead poisoning should be part of the routine pediatric well child care.

High Risk Factors. Situations that should alert a pediatrician to the necessity for screening tests for lead include the following:

•Symptoms such as loss of appetite, abdominal cramps, constipation, anemia, lethargy, or periodic vomiting.

•Children living in housing built before 1978 or in older housing that is being renovated.

•Children living near heavy traffic areas, waste sites, incinerators, or lead smelter plants.

•Children whose parents have lead-related occupations or hobbies.

•Children who suffer from pica or failure to thrive.

Occupational Risks. The risk of lead poisoning in a child of a parent with an occupational lead exposure may be prevented or lessened by good hygiene and avoidance of carrying dust into the home from the work place. The following is a list of occupations with a potential for exposure to lead:

- Lead smelting
- Battery manufacture
- Radiator repair
- Pottery worker
- Automobile service
- Soldering
- Spray painting or paint removal
- Plumbing
- Gasoline refining
- Firing range worker
- Glass manufacture and stained glass hobby

- Printing
- Bridge and tunnel construction
- Die casting

Advice to Parents. Preventive measures to be taken by parents involve lead paint, soil, drinking water, dishware and canned food, and nutrition.

Lead Paint. 1. Check the home inside and out for peeling paint and test paint chips for lead by using a do-it-yourself kit or by contacting the county or state health department for a laboratory referral. Home test kits are sold by:

Frandon Enterprises, 511 N. 48th St., Seattle, WA 98103, Tel. 1-800-359-9000

HybriBet Systems, Inc., P.O. GBHox 1210, Framingham, MA 01701, Tel. 1-800-262-LEAD

2. Prevent children from eating lead-contaminated dust in the home by wet mopping floors, washing toys, and washing the hands before meals.

3. Don't attempt to remove lead paint yourself. Regular vacuums may spread the dust. Scraping, sanding, or torching paint is dangerous since the dust or vaporized lead paint is easily inhaled.

Contact the Division of Environmental Health in the State Department of Public Health for guidelines that should be followed in removing lead paint.

Soil. Soil is contaminated with lead from paint washed off buildings, automobile exhaust, and industrial plants.

1. Provide the child with a covered sandbox.

2. Make sure children wash their hands before they eat.

Drinking Water. The safe standard for lead content of water is 15 ppb (parts per billion). A list of certified testing laboratories may be obtained from the Environmental Protection Agency. If the water is more than 10 to 15 ppb, do the following:

1. Run the water tap for 1 to 2 minutes early morning or until the water temperature is cold, before using for drinking or cooking.

2. Don't use the hot water tap for drinking, cooking, or mixing infant formula. Hot water contains more lead.

3. Some water filters may be advertised to guarantee removal of lead from drinking water. Carbon filters, sand filters and cartridge filters neither remove lead nor prevent corrosion.

Dishware and Canned Food. The lead in the glazes on pottery and china may not be properly fired in manufacture and may leach into food, fruit juices, or coffee. Some china patterns are manufactured with specially formulated glazes, having no lead or cadmium, and are microwave and dishwasher safe. A list of safe china patterns is available in a consumer guide provided by the Environmental Defense Fund (China), 257 Park Ave. South, New York, NY 10010.

Lead solder is no longer used in most tin cans in the United States but it may be present in canned foods from other countries. The FDA has banned the import of some ceramics from Spain, Italy, Japan, Korea, Mexico, Poland, Portugal and Yugoslavia because they contain dangerous amounts of lead.

Some suggestions to reduce the risk of lead exposure from dishware are as follows:

•Don't use pottery and cans to store foods and beverages.

•Don't use china dishes for heating or microwaving food unless they are guaranteed lead-free.

•Beware of imported highly decorated, glossy, multicolored ceramic dishes or mugs. If in doubt, use only for ornamental purposes.

•Don't store liquor in crystal decanters.

•Safe dishes are made of clear glass, undecorated stoneware, or certified low-lead china.

Nutrition. Iron or calcium deficiency promotes lead absorption from the intestine.

•Have your child tested for anemia if you are living in a high risk environment.

•Be sure the diet has sufficient iron and calcium and ask the pediatrician about the necessity for dietary supplements.

COMMUNITY AND PUBLIC HEALTH ROLES

Public health officials work in collaboration with physicians and education, social service and housing agencies that have a role in community efforts to prevent lead exposure and poisoning. Lead poisoning requires a coordinated approach. Patients are diagnosed by doctors and nurses providing routine health care. Local health departments visit high-risk neighborhoods to set up screening clinics. State laboratories arrange for testing of blood samples.

State Departments of Public Health have a Case Registry for reported cases of lead poisoning in children younger than 16 years. A surveillance system collects data on sources of lead and abatement measures, treatment, and patient development, which helps in formulating a public policy regarding lead poisoning in a community.

Communication between local, state, and federal agencies should deal with health, housing, environmental, and children's welfare issues and lead to joint prevention strategies. Community intervention requires to address the following to be successful:

1. Determination of populations at risk for lead exposure.

2. Education of parents, day care providers, and landlords about lead poisoning risks and preventive measures.

3. Arranging for a program of risk abatement in the community and particularly in old, high-risk housing neighborhoods.

Guidelines for the Detection and Management of Lead Poisoning, provided by the Illinois Department of Public Health and other States Agencies for use by Physicians and Health Care Providers, should do much to prevent and provide optimal treatment for this so-called silent epidemic. Lead affects 17 per cent of all American preschool children and approximately 175,000 young children in the State of Illinois.

The morbidity and mortality from acute encephalopathy due to high levels of lead absorption have been reduced remarkably by improved diagnostic tests and improved chelation treatment. Efforts are now being directed to the elimination of exposures to lower doses of lead. Low lead blood levels have been found to result in subtle but none the less serious health problems in young children.

To quote the warning of Rene Dubos, scientist and philosopher, more than 20 years ago: "The problem of lead poisoning is so well-defined, so neatly packaged with both causes and cures known, that if we don't eliminate this social crime, our society deserves all the disasters that have been forecast for it."

Agency for Toxic Substances and Disease Registry, Public Health Service, U.S. Department of Health and Human Services: The nature and extent of lead poisoning in children in the United States. A Report to Congress, 1988. *This report is a comprehensive review of the sources and effects of lead poisoning in childhood.*

Chisolm JJJr. Increased Lead Absorption and Lead Poisoning (Plumbism). In: Behrman RE (ed): Nelson Textbook of Pediatrics, 14th edition. Philadelphia, WB Saunders, 1992,pp 1788-91. *A pediatric expert's account of the diagnosis and management of lead poisoning in children.*

Durback LF, Wedin GP, Seidler DE. Management of lead foreign body ingestion. Clin Toxicol 27: 173, 1989. *A lead muzzle ball swallowed by a 9 year old girl and passed in the stools within 2 weeks without ill effects.*

Huseman CA, Varma MM, Angle CR. Neuroendocrine effects of toxic and low blood lead levels in children. Pediatrics 90:186,1992. *This current publication studies aspects of human growth hormone secretion in children with elevated blood lead levels and lead-induced short stature.*

Illinois Department of Public Health. Guidelines for the Detection and Management of Lead Poisoning for Physicians and Health Care Providers. April 1992. *This report was developed with the assistance of the Medical Advisory Committee for the Childhood Lead Poisoning Prevention Program, the Illinois State Medical*

Society, the Illinois Chapter of the American Academy of Pediatrics, and the Illinois Academy of Family Physicians. It provides information on the new Federal guidelines for determining lead poisoning at lower levels of blood lead and contains updated information on the medical management and treatment of children with lead poisoning.

Louria DB. Trace Metal Poisoning. In: Wyngaarden JB, Smith LH Jr, Bennett JC (eds), Cecil Textbook of Medicine, Philadelphia, WB Saunders, 1992, pp2361-63. *A medical internist's account of lead poisoning with emphasis on adults.*

Millichap JG (ed). Progress in Pediatric Neurology. Chicago, PNB Publisher, 1991, pp441-444. *A review and commentary on recent scientific articles concerning low dose lead exposure and harmful effects on learning in children.*

Myers SL. New York Lead-Test Results, Meant to Reassure, Do the Opposite. New York Times Sunday, Sept 6, 1992; sect 1: 49. *The tests found that soil near the Williamsburg, Brooklyn and Manhattan bridges contained concentrations of lead that far exceeded levels considered safe. A sandblasting crew had spewed lead-contaminated dust, grit and paint chips from the bridge onto streets, playgrounds, and homes.*

Whanger PD. Factors Affecting the Metabolism of Nonessential Metals in Food. In: Hathcock JN (ed), Nutritional Toxicology, vol 1, New York, Academic Press, 1982, pp185-195. *An excellent account of various scientific studies of lead content of food in the diet and nutritional factors that alter lead absorption and excretion.*

CHAPTER 2

TRACE METAL POISONING

> ***"Is there poison in your mouth?"***
> ***"60 Minutes" CBS, Dec 16, 1990.***

In a small percentage of dental patients with hypersensitivity to mercury, there is a potential risk in the use of mercury amalgam.

MERCURY

SOURCES. Mercury and its ore, cinnabar (mercuric sulfide), have been used for at least 2000 years. Early medical prescriptions included mercury as an aphrodisiac and a treatment for syphilis and leprosy. It was also used as a cathartic, teething powder, topical antiseptic, anthelmintic, and diuretic. The

Chinese believed that cinnabar was a medicine which could prolong life, and several emperors are reported to have died looking for immortality by ingesting mercury.

At present its medicinal uses are minimal but more than 60 occupations involve mercury exposure. These include the manufacture of pesticides, insecticides, and fungicides; chloralkali industries; mercury-containing instruments, lamps, neon lights, batteries, paper and pulp manufacturing, paint, dye, electrical equipment, and jewelry; and amalgamation and dentistry. The use of mercury in dental offices has lessened substantially in recent years.

In addition to occupational or industrial exposure, poisoning has resulted from contamination of grains in agriculture and the use of organomercurial compounds as bactericide-fungicide agents. The accidental or intentional ingestion or injection of mercury or mercury-containing compounds also accounts for some cases of poisoning. Fish contaminated with mercury from industrial wastes and agricultural insecticides has become a source of concern in the Midwest inland lakes of the United States. Recent tests of lake water by the Environmental Protection Agency were positive for mercury in 90 percent of samples from 380 different sources.

MERCURY IN FOODS. Organomercurial insecticides are sprayed on fruits and vegetables, including strawberries, peaches, apples, cherries, peas, potatoes, and tomatoes. Seed dressings containing mercury are applied to barley, beans, corn, oats, peanuts, rice, rye, safflower, soybeans, sugarbeets, and wheat. Over 100 pesticide preparations contain mercurials. Poisoning is commonly associated with the inadvertent or uninformed misuse of mercury-containing agricultural preparations.

Mercury is found in organic and inorganic forms in various foods and food products. The Food and Drug Administration has set the limit of mercury content of food at 50 ppb. The estimated average daily intake of mercury in food by Americans is 12 mcg. The mean mercury contents (ppb) of various fruits, garden crops, grains, animal meats, and fish are shown in Table 2.1.

TABLE 2.1. Mercury Content of Various Foods.

Mercury (ppb)	*Food Item*
10 - 50	fruits, vegetables, grain, plant leaves
10 - 200	chicken, pork, lamb, and beef
100 - 600	fish

A significant elevation in these values points to mercury contamination of a part of the ecosystem. Some environmental groups stress the dangers of mercury-contaminated fish in inland lakes and call for more stringent industrial emission standards and regular consumption advisories. State Departments of Natural Resources publish health guides for people who eat sport fish and list contaminated rivers and lakes.

METABOLISM OF MERCURY. The biological effects, tissue distribution, and toxicity of mercury are dependent on the form in which it is absorbed. The human adult body contains about 12 mg mercury, 70 percent in fat and muscle tissues. Mercury has a strong affinity for sulfhydryl, amine, phosphoryl, and carboxyl groups and inactivates a wide variety of enzymes. Exposure to mercury occurs in metallic, inorganic, and organic forms.

Metallic mercury vaporizes with gentle heating, and it is not surprising to find mercury present in all organisms. Up to 10 per cent of dental offices have been found to have excessive mercury vapor levels. The slow intraoral leakage of mercury from dental amalgams is also a concern. *Inorganic mercury* compounds differ in their effects on biological systems. Mercuric sulfide (cinnabar), mercuric chloride (corrosive sublimate), and mercurous chloride (calomel) are relatively nontoxic because of their low solubility and low biological availability. If ingested in large quantities, however, these compounds may cause gastrointestinal symptoms and kidney injury. The mercuric salt is more toxic than mercurous chloride.

Organomercurials include phenyl and methoxy-ethyl mercury salts. They are used as diuretics and fungicides, and have relatively low toxicity, mainly affecting the kidney. Methylmercury, a short-chain alkyl organic mercury compound, is much more toxic than ethyl, diethyl, and other mercury compounds when ingested chronically.

The reasons for the toxicity of methylmercury are as follows:

•Absorption of methylmercury from the intestine is greater than 90 percent compared to 2-50 percent for inorganic mercury.

•Methylmercury is more stable than other organic mercury compounds when absorbed in the body and it circulates unchanged in the blood.

•The biological half-life is 2 to 3 months in man and more than 6 months in fish. Unlike inorganic mercuric compounds, methylmercury remains in the body for extended periods.

•Methylmercury penetrates the blood-brain barrier and 10 percent accumulates in the brain, causing irreversible central nervous system damage.

•Methylmercury penetrates the placenta, accumulating in the fetus, and it is transmitted to newborn infants through the mother's milk, causing brain damage.

Interaction with Essential Nutrients. Mercury affects the metabolism of a number of essential nutrients, including vitamin E, ascorbic acid, zinc, copper, and selenium. These interactions vary with the chemical form of mercury. Methylmercury affects the metabolism of iron, magnesium, and manganese, whereas inorganic mercury has no influence. The protein status of animals affects their ability to resist the toxicity of mercury.

Selenium has been reported to alleviate the toxicity of both organic and inorganic mercury. Sensitivity to mercury- based paints and sprays, as manifested by skin rash, incoordination, and memory loss, was markedly reduced in one patient after adding selenium supplements to her diet. It is difficult to assess the toxicity of mercury in seafoods since they are high in selenium which may counteract the adverse effects.

Pyridoxine (vitamin B_6) can increase the toxicity of mercury and is an example of an essential nutrient causing an adverse effect when administered in excess.

Bioaccumulation in the Food Chain. At each step of the food chain, starting with bacteria and other microbes and ending with fish and fish-eating birds and animals, there is a biological concentration of mercury. The amount of mercury found in fish may be 3000 times the original concentration in the contaminated water. Since methylmercury is 1000 times more soluble in fats than in water, it concentrates in muscle and brain tissue and favors bioaccumulation.

Mercury can also be transferred through the food chain from mercurial treated seed to seed-eating wild birds and from the birds to carnivorous animals. When game birds consume contaminated seeds, methylmercury can accumulate in tissue at levels higher than those accepted as safe for human consumption.

INCIDENCE AND EPIDEMIOLOGY. An estimated 2000 persons have been poisoned by mercury during the last two centuries, with more than 100 deaths, and 6,500 were poisoned since 1972, with more than 400 deaths, all in Iraq. The poisonings in Iraq resulted from the consumption of grains treated with organomercurials. The majority of deaths from mercury have been attributed to this source.

Examples of large scale outbreaks of methylmercury poisoning date back to 1950, when fishermen and their families around Minamata Bay in Japan were stricken with a mysterious neurological disease. The source of poisoning was the consumption of fish and shellfish contaminated with methylmercury derived from materials discharged into the bay from vinyl chloride and acetaldehyde manufacturing plants.

Until the 1960s, mercury discharged into waterways was thought to remain stable or to form relatively harmless compounds with other elements. When fish downstream from pulp and paper mills were found to contain methylmercury, scientists discovered that microorganisms in the water and in the digestive tracts of animals were responsible for the methylation of mercury. All forms of mercury can be converted to methylmercury and are potentially hazardous as food contaminants.

In 1969, the consumption of pork by a family in New Mexico resulted in the hospitalization of 4 children suffering from ataxia, impaired vision, and coma, and irreversible damage to the central nervous system. The patients' blood revealed contamination with mercury (2-3 ppm), the pork liver contained 27 ppm, and the waste seed grain that had been used to feed the hog had 32 ppm derived from methlmercury fungicide. Of 18 hogs owned by the family and fed the contaminated grain, 14 became ataxic and blind and 12 died.

The outbreak of methylmercury poisoning in Iraq occurred as the result of eating homemade bread prepared from wheat treated with fungicide and intended for planting purposes only. Flour made from this treated grain contained 8 ppm alkylmercury. The lowest threshold body burden of methylmercury (25 mg) was associated with the onset of numbness in the fingers and toes. Ataxia began with 55 mg, speech problems at 90 mg, deafness at 170 mg, and death occurred at about 200 mg methylmercury body content.

CLINICAL MANIFESTATIONS. Exposure to high concentrations of mercury vapor may cause fever, chills, cough, chest pain, hemoptysis and pulmonary irritation or pneumonitis. Nausea, vomiting, diarrhea, abdominal pain, and headache are additional symptoms. Inhaled elemental mercury is absorbed through the lung alveoli and may affect the brain.

Micromercurialism. With mild exposure the symptoms are subtle and diagnosis is difficult. Insomnia, nervousness, mild tremor, impaired judgement, fatigue, loss of sexual drive, and depression are symptoms often mistakenly ascribed to psychogenic causes. As the toxicity increases, the patient develops a metallic taste, abdominal cramps, diarrhea, and skin rash.

More advanced stages of chronic mercury poisoning are manifested by a wide array of serious neurological problems, including persistent tremors of the extremities, tongue and lips; a progressive cerebellar syndrome, with ataxia of gait, intention tremor, and dysarthria; delusions and hallucinations; and a polyneuropathy, with sensory impairments of the extremities, including paresthesias and acrodynia. Damage to the kidneys may result in the nephrotic syndrome, with proteinuria, edema, anuria, and uremia. The gums may become swollen and have a blue line around the tooth margins.

ACRODYNIA. Also known as Pink Disease, Swift Disease, Feer Disease, Erythredema, or Dermato-polyneuritis. Acrodynia, Greek for "painful extremities", is a syndrome of chronic mercury poisoning in infants and young children that may be described as a picture of extreme and persistent misery. There is a history of repeated contact with or ingestion of mercury in house products such as paints, wallpapers, teething powders, vermifuges, and diaper rinses. A broken thermometer and vaporization of mercury spilled on a floor radiator in a Canadian home was the cause in one of several cases treated personally by the author. A sensitization to mercury may be involved in etiology, and the interval between exposure and onset of symptoms has varied from 1 week to several months.

Unacceptable levels of mercury vapor were recorded not only in incubators but in the room atmosphere of special care baby units during a 1985 survey of health regions in England. The breakage of clinical glass thermometers and spill of mercury were responsible for this air contamination and significant risk of poisoning. The scale of the problem and potential risk could be appreciated by a report of 1600 broken thermometers over a 6-month period at a Glasgow Children's Hospital. The toxic mercury vapor is inhaled or absorbed through the skin. There are no reports of breakage of a thermometer in the mouth causing poisoning from swallowed or aspirated mercury. Elemental mercury is not toxic when ingested.

Broken barometers in the home and sphygmomanometers in doctor's offices are additional sources of mercury vapor poisoning. Spilled mercury gravitates to cracks in the floor and into the pile of carpets. Vacuuming a contaminated area may facilitate the spread of mercury vapor throughout the house, and warm air from heating ducts and vents may enhance volatilization. Since mercury vapor concentration is likely to be highest near the floor, toddlers may be at greater risk of poisoning than adults.

Clinical Manifestations. The child becomes listless, restless, and irritable. The tips of the fingers, toes, and nose acquire a pinkish color, a distinctive feature of the disease, and generalized transient skin rashes are a frequent occurrence. The hands and feet are swollen and the skin of the palms and soles sheds in scales or sheets. Constant itching, pain, and perspiration lead to a sustained wringing and rubbing of the hands and feet, with the development of ulcers and occasionally, gangrene of fingers and toes.

The gums become inflamed and swollen, salivation is pronounced, and the appetite is lost. The face is buried in the bed linen to shield the eyes from light and photophobia. The hair and nails frequently fall out. Laxity of ligaments and reduced muscle tone are associated with unusual postures, and the child has no desire to sit or walk. The tendon reflexes are depressed or lost. The child with acrodynia is always uncomfortable and irritable and appears apathetic and melancholic.

Treatment and Prevention. Removal of the source of mercury, antidotes, and supportive measures are the key stones of therapy. Mercurial drugs should be avoided in pediatric practice, and the physician should be alert to other sources of mercury in household products and especially in food contaminated by agricultural and industrial mercurials.

BAL is an effective antidote but L-Penicillamine given orally is sometimes preferred. Analgesics for pain, nourishing foods containing protein, minerals, and vitamins, intravenous fluids to correct dehydration, and antibiotics for secondary infections are some of the supportive treatments required. The natural course of acrodynia is prolonged, extending for several months to a year, and there are varying grades of severity.

MINAMATA DISEASE. This form of mercury poisoning that occurred among adults and children living around Minamata Bay, Japan, during 1953 to 1966, is symbolic of the tragic health risks of industrial pollution of water. The source was methylmercury absorbed by eating contaminated fish and shellfish. Congenital cases resulted from placental transfer of the poison from the pregnant mothers who had eaten fish. Infants were born with microcephaly and cerebral atrophy. They were retarded in motor and mental development, and exhibited incoordination, tremors, seizures, swallowing and speech disturbances, deafness, and visual impairment. Older children and adults suffered from constriction of the visual fields, deafness, ataxia, tremors, and sensory loss. They were permanently incapacitated.

PREVENTION OF MERCURY POISONING. Prevention is paramount because brain damage resulting from exposure is irreversible. Public health considerations include the following:

- Prevent mercury-treated grain from inadvertent entry to food chain.
- Educate farmers to cover all seeds with soil, so that wild game birds are denied access.
- Ban disposal of industrial mercurial wastes in waterways.

•Test inland lakes and other fisheries for mercury and especially methylmercury, and issue timely warnings and fishing regulations.

•Reduce the mercury content of poultry and seafoods, which account for nearly all the mercury intake of Americans.

•Avoid mercury exposure from agricultural chemicals, occupational sources, dental amalgams and offices, medicines, and household products.

•Remove mercury thermometers from neonatal units and other Children's Hospital wards and substitute with a safer alternative.

Agocs MM, Etzel RA, Parrish RG et al. Mercury exposure from interior latex paint. N Engl J Med 323:1096, 1990.

Blumenthal I. Should we ban the mercury thermometer? Discussion paper. J R Coll Physicians 85: 553, 1992.

Clarkson TW. Mercury-an element of mystery. N Engl J Med 323:1137, 1990.

D'Itri PA, D'Itri FM. Mercury Contamination: A Human Tragedy. New York, Wiley, 1977.

Fung YK, Molvar MP. Toxicity of mercury from dental environment and from amalgam restorations. Clin Toxicol 30: 49, 1992.

Harada Y, Moriyama H. Congenital Minamata disease. Bull Inst Constitut Med Kumamoto Univ 26: 1, 1976.

Louria DB. Trace Metal Poisoning. In: Wyngaarden JB, Smith LHJr, Bennett JC. (eds), Cecil Textbook of Medicine. Philadelphia, WB Saunders, 1992, pp2363-64.

Mahaffey KR, Corneliussen PE, Jelinek CF, Fiorino JA. Heavy metal exposure from foods. Environ Health Perspect 12: 63, 1975.

Taueg C, Sanfilppo DJ, Rowens B et al. Acute and chronic poisoning from residential exposures to elemental mercury - Michigan, 1989-1990. Clin Toxicol 30: 63, 1992.

Warkany J, Hubbard DM. Acrodynia and mercury. J. Pediat 42: 365, 1953.

Whanger PD. Factors Affecting the Metabolism of Nonessential Metals in Food. In: Hathcock JN (ed), Nutritional Toxicology vol 1, New York, Academic Press, 1982, pp174-184.

ARSENIC

SOURCES. Arsenic is ubiquitous and is found in high concentrations in some well water. Elemental arsenic occurs in nature as a brittle metal and is nontoxic. The toxic forms of arsenic are the pentavalent and trivalent salts, and arsine gas. Arsenic in foods is usually pentavalent and is rapidly excreted. Trivalent arsenic, which is more toxic, accumulates in the body more readily than the pentavalent form. Arsine gas, the most toxic form of arsenic, is formed by the hydrolysis of metallic arsenide or the action of acids on arsenical compounds. It is manufactured in the electronics industry and in metal refining, and it is a source of poisoning when liberated in sewage plants.

Exposure to toxic levels of arsenic may occur in certain occupations: glass, pigment, textile, tanning, bronze-plating and metal alloy industries, and in wood preservation. The burning of arsenate-treated wood is a potential hazard. Farmers are in contact with arsenic in herbicides, insecticides, rodenticides, and in veterinary medicines. Poisoning also results from the ingestion of certain herbal preparations, arsenic-containing medicines, and moonshine whiskey. Pregnant mothers who received arsenical injections for the treatment of venereal disease could expose their infants through breast milk.

In 1987, an episode of acute massive arsenic intoxication involving 718 persons in Argentina was traced to the adulteration of minced meat with sodium arsenite. Vandals had broken into a butcher's shop and poured an acaricide, a sodium arsenite solution of mite insecticide, over 200 kg of meat.

ARSENIC IN FOODS. Meat, fish, and poultry contain the greatest quantities of arsenic, and shellfish are especially contaminated. Cow's milk has an average of 30-60 ppb and up to 1500 ppb in milk from cows grazing in arsenic-contaminated fields. Organic compounds such as arsanilic acid, used as growth stimulants in pigs and poultry, are rapidly excreted and when fed in recommended amounts, do not accumulate excessively in meat animals. The average daily intake of arsenic for Americans is estimated at about 10 mcg.

CLINICAL MANIFESTATIONS. Arsine gas poisoning is acute in onset and frequently fatal. All systems of the body are affected. Presenting symptoms include fever, headache, muscle and abdominal pains, nausea, vomiting, diarrhea, and dysuria. Hemolytic anemia, hemoglobinuria, and renal failure are often accompanied by signs of vascular collapse, myocardial damage, and encephalopathy. Patients who recover from the acute episode may suffer from chronic kidney failure.

Arsenic Ingestion. The early symptoms of arsenic food poisoning are similar to those at the onset of arsine inhalation but they are much less dramatic and usually insidious and subtle. A metallic taste, often associated with a garlic odor to the breath, is not pathognomonic and is observed with other trace metal intoxications, including selenium.

Other manifestations occurring in the first week include jaundice, enlarged liver, heart disease, lung edema, kidney failure, psychosis and encephalopathy. Headache and irritability become worse and confusion, delusions, hallucinations, seizures, and optic neuritis may develop.

A symmetric polyneuropathy is the most prominent sign after the first week of illness. The patient first complains of a burning sensation in a stocking and glove distribution and later develops severe weakness with absent tendon reflexes. Both sensory and motor nerve involvements are apparent.

Chronic poisoning is characterized by skin and nail lesions, notably pigmentation (arsenic melanosis), thickening of the palms and soles (hyperkeratosis), and transverse white bands in the nails (Aldrich-Mees lines). Depigmentation of the skin and hair loss may also occur. Skin cancers appear in 5 to 10 percent of patients after latent periods of 5 to 25 years. The most common cause of arsenic-related skin cancers in the United States was formerly the medicinal use of Fowler's solution (potassium arsenite), which is now obsolete, and occupational exposure is currently invoked. Lung and liver cancers have also been correlated with exposure to arsenic trioxide in gold and tin miners, smelter workers, and laborers in vineyards and sheep-dip factories.

INCIDENCE. Arsenic was the popular poisoning agent of the Middle Ages and was favored by felons until the early 1900s. It was easily obtained, had little taste, and could be administered to the unwary victim in food without detection. The alertness of physicians in recognizing early signs of arsenic poisoning, laws prohibiting its use in embalming solutions, and chemical tests for minute quantities have greatly discouraged the use of this agent for this purpose.

The incidence of accidental poisoning with arsenic has also diminished in recent times because of its limited application as a medicine. However, arsenic is still employed in agricultural insecticides and pesticides. Among the heavy metals, arsenic ranks second to lead as a cause of death from accidental poisoning in children. Occupational hazards account for chronic arsenic poisoning in adults.

Mechanism of Action. All arsenicals exert their toxicity by reacting with sulfhydryl groups in cells. Enzyme systems essential to cellular metabolism are inhibited. Trivalent organic arsenicals, the most toxic form, are more potent inhibitors of sulfhydryl enzymes than the less toxic inorganic arsenites. The greatest inactivation of these enzymes by arsenicals is caused by the blistering agent, lewisite, used in warfare.

DIAGNOSIS. Arsenic can be measured in blood, urine, hair, or nails by absorption spectrophotometry or neutron activation techniques. A qualitative urine test (Gutzeit test) is also available.

TREATMENT. Dimercaprol (BAL) given within 24 hours of exposure is the treatment of choice.

Exchange transfusion, dialysis, or penicillamine are also recommended. The neuropathy and kidney failure are sometimes refractory to treatment.

PREVENTION. Most arsenic poisoning can be avoided by taking appropriate precautions in those occupations known to be at risk. Well water should be examined for contamination. Herbal preparations of undetermined composition should be obtained only from reliable sources. Physicians must be alert to the early manifestations of arsenic poisoning so that treatment may be prescribed promptly.

Harvey SC. Heavy Metals. In: Goodman LS and Gilman A (eds), The Pharmacological Basis of Therapeutics, 3rd ed, New York, Macmillan, 1965, pp944-951.

Roses OE, Garcia Fernandez JC, Villaamil EC et al. Mass poisoning by sodium arsenite. Clin Toxicol 29: 20 1991.

Schoolmeester WL, White DR. Arsenic poisoning. South Med J 73: 198, 1980. *A review with more than 100 references and 10 case reports.*

Wu MM, Kuo TL, Hwang YH, Chen CJ. Dose response relation between arsenic concentration in well water and mortality from cancers and vascular diseases. Am J Epidemiol 130: 1123, 1989. *An epidemiological study with 53 references.*

CADMIUM

SOURCES. Cadmium occurs in nature as an inorganic form, principally as the sulfide, and is bound to organic compounds in plants and animal tissues. The lower the soil pH, the greater the uptake of cadmium in plants. Agricultural practices and use of sludge from sewage plants as a fertilizer and contaminated pesticides may increase the cadmium content of foods. Humans may be exposed to unusually high levels of cadmium in certain industrial occupations or via polluted food and water and industrial wastes. People who prepare or store food and water in galvanized containers are at risk.

Occupations at risk for cadmium poisoning include the manufacture of electrical conductors, electroplating, alloys, zinc refining, soldering, engraving, ceramics, pigments, dentistry, plastics, storage batteries; photographic, rubber, and aircraft industries; and smelting and metal-processing industries.

CADMIUM CONTENT OF FOODS. Foods which contain high levels of cadmium include oysters, clams, liver, and kidney. The cadmium content of food classes is highest for leafy vegetables, potatoes and fruits (average, 47 ppb), and lowest for dairy products and beverages (5 ppb) and for meat, fish, and poultry (9 ppb). The major food groups contributing cadmium as a percentage of the total daily consumption are grains and cereals, 23 per cent; fruits and leafy vegetables, 18 per cent; and potatoes, 18 per cent. The estimated total daily intake of cadmium from food for Americans is about 50 mcg.

METABOLISM. The absorption of cadmium is very low, but once accumulated in the tissues, it remains and excretion is minimal. Deposited chiefly in the kidney, the biological half-life of cadmium may be more than 30 years. The prevention of exposure and tissue accumulation is important to avoid kidney damage, particularly in infancy and early childhood. One third of the cadmium in the adult body has been absorbed in the first few years of life.

The amount of cadmium in the diet needed to cause toxicity is estimated at 300 mcg per day, about six times the current average daily intake. Although the risks of poisoning from ingestion of cadmium in food seem small, a number of factors are known to influence the toxicity, and a safe threshold level of cadmium in food does not apply in all circumstances.

Interactions with proteins, vitamins, and minerals affect the toxicity of cadmium. A low-protein intake and calcium and vitamin D deficiencies exacerbate the adverse effect of cadmium on growth and may induce abnormal spinal curvature and osteomalacia.

The quality of protein in the diet may also be a factor. An excess of cysteine containing protein, vitamin C, and the minerals, zinc, iron, copper, and selenium, has a protective effect and decreases the toxicity of cadmium, whereas deficiencies of protein, minerals, and vitamin D increase the sensitivity to cadmium toxicity.

Cadmium also disrupts the metabolism of copper and results in lowering of plasma ceruloplasmin levels. Pyridoxine supplements may exacerbate cadmium toxicity.

CLINICAL MANIFESTATIONS. *Acute intoxication* after ingestion of 5 gm cadmium, sufficient to commit suicide, caused damage to liver and kidneys and heart irregularities. The levels of cadmium in tissues at autopsy were highest in the liver and kidney (80 ppm), lower in the heart (10 ppm), and least in the brain (0.5 ppm). The accidental ingestion of smaller amounts results in gastroenteritis which lasts for less than 24 hours. Exposure to cadmium fumes causes cough, wheezing, and lung edema.

Chronic poisoning induces proteinuria and kidney damage and is rarely fatal. Industrial aerosol exposure to cadmium for periods greater than 10 years has caused emphysema and olfactory nerve damage, with loss of the sense of smell.

Itai-itai(ouch-ouch)disease affected multiparous Japanese women, ages 40 to 70, who lived in industrial mining areas where cadmium containing waste in sea and river water was used for irrigating rice and for household consumption. Symptoms coincident with kidney damage included severe pains in the back and joints, waddling gait, osteomalacia, skeletal deformities, and bone fractures.

PREVENTION. There is no specific treatment for cadmium poisoning and prevention by avoidance of exposure is all important. A diet high in protein and supplemented with vitamin C and iron may decrease the occupational risks of toxicity in workers exposed to high levels of cadmium.

Anke M, Schneider H (eds). Kadmium Symp. 1979, pp349. *The report of an international symposium on cadmium.*

Brenner I. Cadmium toxicity. World Rev Nutr Diet 32: 165,1978.

Fox, MRS. Effect of essential minerals on cadmium toxicity: A review. J Food Sci 38: 321, 1974.

Lucier GW, Hook GER (eds). Cadmium. Environ Health Perspect 28: 1-112, 1979. *A complete issue devoted to various aspects of cadmium , including metabolism and nutritional relationships.*

Webb M (ed). Chemistry, biochemistry and biology of cadmium. Top Environ Health 2: 465, 1979.

Whanger PD. Factors affecting the metabolism of nonessential metals in food. In: Hathcock JN (ed). Nutritional Toxicology vol 1, New York, Academic Press, 1982, pp164-174.

THALLIUM

SOURCES. Thallium was formerly a component of rodenticides, pesticides, and insecticides, common sources of poisoning that have been largely discontinued. Occupational hazards of exposure include the manufacture of optical lenses, jewelry, low-temperature thermometers, semiconductors, dyes and pigments, scintillation counters, and fireworks. Thallium is used in alloys and is a by-product of lead and zinc production. It can cause toxicity when inhaled, ingested, or absorbed through the skin. A strong affinity for sulfhydryl groups results in interference with enzyme systems.

FOOD CONTENT. The thallium content of food estimates have been sparse and have ranged from nondetectable to 140 ppb in vegetables and bread. The daily intake of thallium in the diet is less than 2 mcg.

CLINICAL MANIFESTATIONS. *Acute poisoning* causes gastrointestinal distress, weakness, confusion, seizures, and coma. *Subacute and chronic thallium intoxications* are characterized by a painful peripheral neuropathy and loss of scalp hair. The predominantly motor paralysis mimics Guillain-Barre syndrome, but the striking total alopecia of the head and associated abdominal pain are suggestive of thallium toxicity. The diagnosis may be confirmed by qualitative and quantitative tests for thallium in the urine.

TREATMENT AND PROGNOSIS. Hemodialysis removes half the body content of thallium, potassium administration displaces thallium from inside cells, and prussian blue or activated charcoal given orally adsorbs charcoal in the intestine. Barbiturates exacerbate the symptoms and should be avoided. Ten percent of acute cases are fatal and 30 per cent of all poisonings leave residual effects, including neuropathy, ataxia, impaired vision, dementia, and myoclonic seizures.

Wainwright AP, Kox WJ, House IM et al. Clinical features and therapy of acute thallium poisoning. Q J Med 69: 939, 1988.

ALUMINUM

SOURCES. Tap water having high concentrations of aluminum is a common cause of dementia following repeated dialyses. In some cases aluminum sulfate has been added to the water supply to remove organic materials. Aluminum-containing gels administered by mouth to reduce phosphate levels may cause encephalopathy in children suffering from renal failure. Occupational hazards involving aluminum aerosol exposure may cause poisoning in welders, bauxite smelters, and pottery or explosive manufacturers. Aluminum pots used in cooking will increase exposure to aluminum in food.

FOOD CONTENT. Aluminum content of foods of plant origin is 100 times that of food derived from animals and ranges from 10 to 30 ppm, depending on the soil aluminum content. The total dietary intake of aluminum by humans varies from 18 to 36 mg/day. It is absorbed from the intestine very slowly and is toxicologically inert, except when the intake is augmented by ingestion of aluminum hydroxide gels and especially in patients with kidney disease and delayed excretion.

CLINICAL MANIFESTATIONS. The majority of cases of aluminum poisoning occur as dialysis encephalopathy in patients on hemodialysis and peritoneal dialysis. The intravenous administration of nutritional solutions containing aluminum may also result in poisoning.

Early manifestations of aluminum-induced dialysis encephalopathy include malaise, memory loss, and speech disturbance. These are followed by myoclonus, somnolence, and dementia. The electroencephalogram shows characteristic abnormal slowing, with bursts of delta and high voltage, symmetric spikes.

Mild forms of encephalopathy in chronic dialysis patients are recognized and are characterized by cognitive and motor deficits, weakness, and mild myoclonus. Some patients develop severe bone and muscle pain, fractures, anemia, cardiomyopathy, and parathyroid dysfunction.

Alzheimer's disease and amyotrophic lateral sclerosis have been linked with high levels of aluminum in the brain, but a causal relation has not been proven.

Aluminum aerosols in the bauxite industry may cause lung fibrosis and emphysema (Shaver's disease), and smelters develop wheezing (potroom asthma).

TREATMENT. The withdrawal of aluminum-containing medications or change to an aluminum-free dialysis water is the first prerequisite. Deferoxamine treatment, which forms a complex with aluminum, can be beneficial but may temporarily exacerbate the encephalopathy.

PROGNOSIS. Dialysis encephalopathy is frequently lethal, and the mean survival time is 6 months. High levels of aluminum are found in bone, liver, and brain of uremic patients dying of dialysis encephalopathy, but a causal association is not definitely determined. Aluminum is known to inhibit enzymes in the brain which alter neurotransmitter metabolism and may be responsible for changes in mood and cognitive abilities, but results of recent studies are conflicting.

PREVENTION. Patients with renal failure and uremia are particularly susceptible to aluminum poisoning and should be aware of risks of overexposure:

•Nonprescription drugs and antacid-gels that are high in aluminum should be avoided.

•Community water supplies with high aluminum content should not be used for drinking or for dialysis.

•Citrates and the drug, cimetidine increase aluminum absorption and should be used with caution.

•Aluminum pots should not be used in cooking.

Other trace elements with toxicities largely associated with hemodialysis include zinc, copper, cobalt, and nickel.

Arieff A. Aluminum and the pathogenesis of dialysis encephalopathy. Am J Kidney Dis 6: 317-321, 1985.

Bolla KI, Milstien S, Briefel G et al. Dihydropteridine reductase activity: Lack of association with serum aluminum levels and cognitive functioning in patients with end-stage renal disease. Neurology 41: 1806, 1991.

Domingo JL. The use of chelating agents in the treatment of aluminum overload. Clin Toxicol 27: 355, 1989.

Gruskin AB. Aluminum: A pediatric overview. Adv Pediatr 35: 281, 1988.

Masselot JP, Adhemar JP, Jaudon MC et al. Reversible dialysis encephalopathy: role for aluminum containing gels. Lancet 2:1386, 1978.

Rosati G, DeBastiani P, Gilli P et al. Oral aluminum and neuropsychological functioning. J Neurol 223: 251, 1980.

Simon P, Allain P, Ang KS et al. Prevention and treatment of aluminum intoxication in chronic renal failure. Adv Nephrol 14: 439, 1985.

OTHER TOXIC NONESSENTIAL METALS

TIN

The tin content of the average American diet ranges from 1 to 38 mg/day. The essential nature of this mineral is debatable. Differences in intake are dependent on the use of canned foods, with levels as high as 150 mcg/gm reported in foods packed in unlacquered containers. The consumption of canned fruits, vegetables, and juices from unlacquered cans could result in a daily intake of tin of more than 200 mg. In contrast, fresh-frozen and bottled foods contain very little tin.

Acute toxicity has resulted from the ingestion of canned juices or acid punches prepared in tinned vessels. The levels of tin in contaminated foods have ranged from 500 to 2000 mcg/ml. Symptoms of intoxication include nausea, abdominal cramps, diarrhea, and vomiting.

Chronic effects on growth, enzymes, blood hemoglobin, and immune function observed in animals may be due to interactions between tin and essential minerals such as zinc, copper, iron, calcium, and selenium. Elderly individuals and children who routinely consume less than the Recommended Dietary Allowances for zinc, calcium, and other minerals are more susceptible to the adverse effects of high dietary levels of tin on bone and other cell metabolism. Fruits, vegetables, and juices packed in unlacquered cans should be avoided particularly in these age groups, and foods should not be stored in opened cans.

NICKEL

Contact dermatitis may occur in allergic persons exposed to nickel-containing prosthetic joints and heart valves, jewelry, pacemakers, and needles used for intravenous fluids. Nickel is a potent respiratory tract carcinogen, and industrial aerosol exposure to nickel carbonyl causes pneumonitis or metal fume fever.

ANTIMONY

Foods cooked or stored in enamel pots and cans may contain levels of antimony sufficient to cause poisoning. The total daily intake for Americans is estimated at 1 mg. Adverse effects include nausea, vomiting, abdominal pain, muscle and joint pain, liver and kidney dysfunction, and cardiac abnormalities.

Treatment of poisoning from oral ingestion of antimony consists of stomach lavage, and administration of activated charcoal and dimercaprol analogues.

BARIUM

Barium is associated with calcium and strontium in the food chain from plants to animals. The estimated daily intake is 1 mg. Brazil nuts are exceptionally rich in barium. Ingestion of large amounts of barium results in abdominal pain, vomiting, and an increase in peristalsis. A lowering of serum potassium is associated with muscle weakness and cardiac arrhythmias. Treatment consists of potassium administration and forced diuresis to promote the urinary excretion of barium. The radiological use of barium may be followed by an allergic reaction.

BORON

Ingestion of boric acid or absorption from skin applications can result in severe toxic reactions, with nausea, vomiting, diarrhea, anemia, skin rashes, convulsions, delirium, and coma. The mortality rate in infants is 70 percent. Hemodialysis may be lifesaving.

Greger JL, Lane HW. The toxicology of dietary tin, aluminum, and selenium. In: Hathcock JN (ed). Nutritional Toxicology vol II, New York, Academic Press, 1987.

Lauwers LF, Roelants A, Rosseel PM et al. Oral antimony intoxications in man. Crit Care Med 18: 324, 1990. *A report of 4 cases due to eating cake tainted with antimony potassium tartrate.*

Louria DB. Trace metal poisoning. In: Wyngaarden JB, Smith LHJr, Bennett, JC (eds). Cecil Textbook of Medicine. Philadelphia, WB Saunders, 1992.

Locatelli C, Minoia C, Tonini M et al. Human toxicology of boron with special reference to boric acid poisoning. Ital Med Lav 9: 141, 1987.

Sigel H, Sigel A (eds). Metal Ions in Biological Systems, vol 23 & 24. New York, Marcel Dekker, 1988.

CHAPTER 3

ESSENTIAL TRACE MINERAL TOXICITY

"Twenty-two heart attack victims were autopsied and all had heart muscle damage attributable to cobalt salts in bcer."
Canad Med Assoc J 97: 910, 1967.

Essential trace minerals, cobalt, copper, fluorine, iron, manganese, selenium, and zinc, may cause disease either as a result of a deficiency state or when consumption is in excess of normal requirements. In some cases poisoning is a consequence of occupational exposure. In others toxicity results from food additives or adulteration, prescription or nonprescription medicines, or from procedures such as hemodialysis or insertion of prostheses.

While acute poisoning from the ingestion of megadoses of the mineral may permit early diagnosis, the recognition of symptoms and signs of chronic, low-level trace element exposure is often difficult and the interactions between minerals are poorly understood.

COBALT

Between 1964 and 1966, brewers were adding cobalt sulfate to their product as a foam stabilizer. An epidemic of heart disease and cardiomyopathy resulted, often accompanied by pericardial effusion, with 48 fatalities in the United States and Canada. If the ingredient responsible for the foamy head on the beer had been indicated on the label, the physicians who were at first baffled by the disease would have diagnosed the toxicity earlier and prescribed specific therapy. This is a tragic example of the consequences of additives in food, permitted without government scientific approval or declaration on labels, and inadvertently used in quantities toxic to humans.

Workers exposed to cobalt in industry may develop cardiomyopathy or lung disease. Patients with kidney failure on hemodialysis have developed cobalt poisoning from the ingestion of cobalt chloride prescribed for anemia. In addition to cardiomyopathy, this source of toxicity has resulted in nausea and vomiting, peripheral neuropathy, goiter, deafness, and optic atrophy.

COPPER

The daily dietary intake of copper ranges between 1 and 5 mg, of which about 40 per cent is absorbed. A low-molecular-weight metal protein, metallothionein, is involved in regulating copper absorption at high-copper intakes. Increased urinary copper levels can occur with the dietary use of softened water supplies. Inorganic copper salts are used as astringents, deodorants, and antiseptics. If accidentally ingested, toxicity from these soluble salts is manifested as gastrointestinal upset and hemolytic anemia.

Poisoning may also result during hemodialysis, when copper is a component of the dialysis tubing and water with an acid pH is supplied through copper plumbing. Copper is a red blood cell poison, damaging the cell membranes and causing hemolytic anemia and jaundice. Other signs of toxicity include nausea, vomiting, diarrhea, abdominal pain, pancreatitis, and severe muscle pain with myoglobinemia.

The dusts of inorganic copper salts have low toxicity, but workers in vineyards exposed to copper sulfate spray for prolonged periods have developed *vineyard sprayers' lung disease.* Copper fumes inhaled by metal welders may cause eye and skin irritation, metal fume fever, chemical pneumonitis, and disturbances of the central nervous system.

An additional category of copper compounds are the water insoluble organic forms, such as copper naphthenate, used as a fungicide and rot proofing agent for textiles and wood. A family exposed to copper naphthenate used as a fungicide on the foundation of their home developed gastrointestinal symptoms, headache, conjunctivitis, and neuropsychological abnormalities. Despite permanent evacuation from the house, the patients had elevated serum copper levels even 4 years after exposure.

The dangers of copper poisoning may be minimized by the recognition and avoidance of sources of exposure, decontamination, and chelation therapy if systemic toxicity ensues.

An inborn error of copper metabolism associated with excessive absorption and accumulation of copper in the brain, eye, liver, and kidneys results in the neurological and liver syndrome of Wilson's disease. This brain and hepatic degenerative disease is characterized by tremor, dysarthria, dystonia, and dementia. Rapid increases of circulating copper in this condition can cause acute hemolytic anemia. Treatment consists of a low copper diet and penicillamine, a chelating agent, to promote urinary copper excretion.

FLUORINE

Fluoride salts are found in fluorinated water, dental hygiene products, dietary supplements, and in insecticides and rodenticides. Drinking water accounts for 0.5 to 1.5 mg/day and is the largest single source of dietary intake.

In acute ingestion, fluoride acts as a cellular poison. It inhibits glycolytic and other enzyme systems and depresses tissue respiration. A sharp decline in the serum concentration of calcium occurs within 10 minutes and is responsible for heart irregularities and cardiovascular collapse.

Chronic intoxication (*fluorosis*) may occur from 1) drinking water with very high fluoride concentration, 2) hemodialysis, and 3) industrial inhalation exposure. Significant toxicity is unlikely from household dental hygiene products that contain a maximum of 120 mg fluoride per tube. Musculoskeletal and systemic symptoms develop after many years with a fluoride intake exceeding 6-10 mg/day. The acute ingestion of 30-60 mg/kg may be fatal if untreated. Continuous use of water containing more than 2.5 ppm will result in mottling of dental enamel.

Clinical manifestations of chronic toxicity include weight loss, weakness, myalgia, anemia, brittle bones, stiff joints, and calcification of ligaments and tendons.

Treatment varies with the dose and type of poisoning. For ingestions less than 5 mg/kg, milk to relieve gastrointestinal symptoms is sufficient. For larger amounts, antacids or calcium chloride are given to bind or precipitate the fluoride; gastric lavage is recommended to remove the stomach contents; calcium gluconate may be required to correct the hypocalcemia; and intravenous fluids to induce an alkaline diuresis. Cation exchange resins or dialysis may be necessary to reverse a fluoride-induced hyperkalemia. The time to complete recovery may be prolonged but the prognosis is good, if the patient survives more than 24 hours after acute ingestions.

IRON

As few as 10 to 15 ferrous sulfate candy-coated tablets may be fatal if ingested by a child. Doses as low as 60 mg/kg of elemental iron have caused death. Symptoms may occur within thirty to sixty minutes. Four clinical stages of acute iron poisoning have been described:

1. Abdominal pain, vomiting, and diarrhea.
2. *Latent* phase of clinical improvement from 6-24 hours after ingestion, when the patient is relatively asymptomatic.
3. Hepatic and renal shutdown, with cardiovascular collapse.
4. Gastrointestinal strictures and obstruction.

Adults as well as children are at risk for severe gastrointestinal complications after iron overdose. Significant protracted abdominal pain should alert the physician to this diagnosis. Damage to the large bowel can occur, with complete sparing of the stomach and small intestine, if the iron is ingested as an enteric-coated preparation.

Chronic ingestion of iron supplements in the diet or excess meat may predispose to heart attacks, according to a recent report from Finland. In men with a blood ferritin level twice normal, the risk of heart attack was doubled. Women lose iron every month during menstruation and they are less susceptible to heart attacks than men.

Treatment. Gastric lavage should be followed with bicarbonate solution to convert free ferrous salt into poorly absorbed ferrous carbonate. Surgical or GI consultation is advised to identify and treat bleeding sites. Chelation therapy with deferoxamine is indicated with serum iron concentrations greater than 300 mcg/dL. An upper GI series of X-rays is advised 6 weeks after ingestion of excess iron to exclude strictures or obstructions in the bowel.

MANGANESE

Manganese ingestion or contamination of dialysates may result in abdominal pain, liver dysfunction, and pancreatitis. Manganese dioxide aerosol exposure causes *manganic madness* in miners. The concentration of manganese in the basal ganglia and cerebellum accounts for the Parkinsonian-like facies, rigidity, and ataxia. Psychotic behavior may be the dominant feature and is manifested by compulsive singing, laughter, dancing, fighting, and running. The mental aberrations improve after treatment with calcium versenate and L-dopa, but the neurologic abnormalities usually persist.

In a recent report of an 8 year-old girl with a dystonic movement disorder due to manganese poisoning, the symptoms were reversible. The toxicity was dietary in origin, and manganese accumulation in the brain resulted from liver disease and impaired excretion in the bile.

SELENIUM

The amount of selenium in the diet varies with the types of foods eaten and the geographic soil content. Foods high in selenium include grains, pork, fish, chicken, egg yolk, beef, garlic, mushrooms, and radishes. Industrial exposure occurs in the manufacture of pigment, glass, electronics, ceramics, and steel. Toxicity due to selenium fumes is manifested by apathy, lassitude, pallor, cough, nervousness, depression, hair and nail loss, a garlic odor to the breath, and a metallic taste.

Poisoning by excessive ingestion of selenium causes nausea, vomiting, abdominal pain, diarrhea, fatigue, joint pains, hair loss, garlic breath, bronze skin, liver dysfunction, and skin rash. An epidemic of chronic selenium intoxication occurred in China in the 1960s which was attributed to selenium-laden vegetables.

An unproven suggestion that increased selenium intake may modify or prevent human cancer, particularly of the intestinal tract, has promoted the sale of nonprescription selenium supplements, which may lead to an increasing frequency of chronic selenium toxicity.

ZINC

The daily intake of zinc ranges from 5 to 35 mg. Zinc is bound to metallothioneins and is excreted by the urinary and intestinal tracts. It has a strong affinity for red cells and plasma proteins, and high concentr-ations are found in the eye and prostate.

Sources of zinc poisoning include the zinc oxide adhesive plaster used to prevent dialysis coils from unwinding, the water of the dialysis fluid, and galvanized iron pipes or tanks used in plumbing. Zinc poisoning associated with hemodialysis may be prevented by using deionized or distilled water. Welders, smelter workers, and solderers exposed to aerosolized zinc may experience zinc fume fever, with lung dysfunction.

Clinical manifestations of oral or parenteral zinc toxicity include nausea, vomiting, weakness, abdominal pain, and anemia. Severe poisoning results in pancreatitis and renal failure.

The dangers of zinc deficiency are generally greater than those of zinc excess. In the villages of Iran and Turkey, a zinc deficiency syndrome of dwarfism, anemia, and sexual underdevelopment has been related to the habit of geophagia, the eating of earthy substances such as clay. Clinical pictures similar to the zinc-deficient dwarfs in Iran occur in the United States, especially in persons who eat primarily cereal proteins and little meat.

CHROMIUM

The estimated safe and adequate daily dietary intake of chromium varies from 10-60 mcg for infants, 20-120 mcg in young children, and 50-200 mcg in adolescents and adults. An impaired glucose tolerance in malnourished children and in some mild diabetics will respond to chromium supplements. Chromium is contained in some high energy food supplements favored by body building enthusiasts.

Foods of higher chromium content and bioavailability include brewer's yeast, calf's liver, American cheese, and wheat germ. While supplements of 150 mcg/day are nontoxic, a varied diet is the best assurance of an adequate and safe chromium intake.

Chronic toxicity from occupational exposure to dusts containing chromate causes ulceration of the skin, respiratory symptoms and an increased incidence of bronchial cancer. An acute poisoning in an infant who ingested chromate-containing paint pigment caused neurological symptoms of encephalopathy.

Banner WJ, Tong TG. Iron poisoning. Pediatr Clin North Am 33: 393, 1986.

Bencko V, Cikrt M. Manganese: a review of toxicology. J Hyg Epidem Microbiol Immunol 28: 139, 1984.

Bluhm RE, Welch L, Branch RA. Residential exposure to copper naphthenate. Clin Toxicol 30: 99, 1992.

Delves HT. Dietary sources of copper. In: Biological Roles of Copper. Ciba Found Symp 79: 5, 1980.

Fosmire GJ. Zinc toxicity. Am J Clin Nutr 51: 225, 1990.

Millichap JG (ed). Manganese toxicity. Ped Neur Briefs 6; 83: 1992.

Noji EK, Kelen GD. (eds). Manual of Toxicologic Emergencies. Chicago, Year Book Med Publ, 1989.

Smith KT (ed). Trace Minerals In Foods. New York, Marcel Dekker, 1988.

Sunderman FWJr. A review of the metabolism and toxicity of nickel. Ann Clin Lab Sci 7: 377, 1977.

Tenenbein M, Littman C, Stimpson RE. Gastrointestinal pathology in adult iron overdose. Clin Toxicol 28: 311, 1990.

Webster JD, Parker TF, Alfrey A et al. Acute nickel intoxication by dialysis. Ann Intern Med 92:631, 1980.

Yang G, Wang S, Zhou R et al. Endemic selenium intoxication of humans in China. Am J Clin Nutr 37: 872, 1983.

Yolken R, Konecny P, McCarthy P. Acute fluoride poisoning. Pediatrics 58: 90, 1976.

CHAPTER 4

EXCESS VITAMIN TOXICITY

"One swears by wholemeal bread, one by sour milk; vegetarianism is the only road to salvation of some, others insist not only on vegetables alone, but on eating those raw. At one time the only thing that matters is calories; at another time they are crazy about vitamins or about roughage. The scientific truth may be put quite briefly; eat moderately, having an ordinary mixed diet, and don't worry." R. Hutchinson. Newcastle Med J 12: 1932.

Vitamins are essential food substances called coenzymes. They function in small quantities to speed up metabolic reactions. If the quantity of vitamin coenzyme in the diet is deficient, the metabolism of carbohydrate, protein, or fatty substances is disrupted, resulting in an abnormal and sometimes toxic accumulation of chemicals in the body. In excess, vitamins, and especially vitamin A, may act as a poison, adversely affecting cell membranes and leading to damaged intracellular organelles and release of toxic proteolytic enzymes.

Classification. Vitamins can be classified into three main groups:

1) *Fat soluble* Vitamins A, D, E, and K;

2) *Water soluble B Vitamins* : B_1 (thiamine), B_2 (riboflavine), B_3 (niacin), B_6 (pyridoxine), B_{12} (cyanocobalamin), folic acid, pantothenic acid, and biotin; and

3) *Water soluble Vitamin C* (ascorbic acid).

Deficiences and excesses of these vitamins may cause disorders of the nervous system and other body functions. The recommended dietary daily allowances (RDA) of vitamins are listed in Table 4-1. Some persons with a vitamin dependency require 10 to 500 times the normal recommended daily allowances of certain vitamins. In most healthy persons, a normal balanced diet supplies sufficient vitamins, and supplements are probably unnecessary and may be harmful.

Even without supplementation, the diet may be high in vitamins as a result of commercial fortification of foods. Vitamins are added to products to prevent deficiences, to improve their market value, or to act as preservatives. Examples include the highly fortified breakfast cereals and fruit juices, the addition of vitamin D to milk, and the incorporation of vitamins C and E as antioxidants.

With increasing fortification and lack of appropriate controls, the consumption of overfortified food staples might result in excessive exposure and risk of vitamin toxicity. As vitamin consumption increases, a higher incidence of toxicity may be anticipated, particularly from vitamins A and D which are stored in the body. The health benefits of optimal vitamin intake must be reconciled with the risks of inadvertent or overzealous vitamin overdose.

VITAMIN A

The major dietary sources of vitamin A are *retinol,* found in foods of animal origin, and *B-carotene,* a pro-vitamin pigment derived from plants. Vitamin A is also synthesized commercially and is supplied as vitamin supplements or as retinoic acid (Accutane, Tigason) for the treatment of acne or psoriasis. Retinol is the active form of the vitamin; carotene is oxidized and converted to retinol in the intestine.

Carotene is generally nontoxic, and large amounts ingested do not raise the circulating serum level of vitamin A. Persons consuming large quantities of carrots or infants fed pureed, carotene containing vegetables develop *hypercarotenosis,* manifested by a yellow pigmentation of the skin which slowly resolves when the dietary source of carotene is avoided.

Retinol is the potentially toxic form of vitamin A. Livers of animals such as polar bears and large marine fish are the only natural foodstuffs containing sufficient retinol to cause poisoning. Arctic explorers and fishermen have suffered symptoms of acute vitamin A intoxication after eating generous portions of these livers which may contain up to 100,000 IU (30,000 mcg retinol).

VITAMIN A VALUE OF DIETS. Compared to retinol, dietary carotenoid provitamins are poorly absorbed in the intestine and have one-sixth or less vitamin A activity. In 1967, a FAO/WHO (Food and Agriculture Organization/World Health Organization) Expert Committee abandoned the term "International Unit (IU)" in favor of "Retinol Equivalent (mcg RE)." The Committee on Recommended Dietary Allowances (RDA) of the National Research Council also approved this change and have expressed the RDAs of vitamin A as retinol equivalents in their revised 1980-89 reports.

The vitamin A value of diets must indicate the percentage derived from retinol and that from carotenoids in plants. Expressed as retinol equivalents (RE) the vitamin A activity of the diet can be calculated from the following:

1 retinol equivalent = 1 mcg retinol = 3.33 IU
1 RE = 6 mcg B-carotene
1 RE = 12 mcg other carotenoids
= 3.33 IU activity as retinol
= 10 IU activity as carotene

Or 1 International Unit = 0.3 mcg retinol
= 0.6 mcg B-carotene

Foods in the United States are estimated to contain about half the total vitamin A activity as retinol and half as provitamin A carotenoids. The adult recommended daily allowance of 5000 IU (1000 mcg RE) is therefore composed of 2500 IU (750 mcg RE) as retinol and 2500 IU (250 mcg RE) as B-carotene.

The recommended daily allowance for infants is based on the retinol content of human milk (49 mcg/100 ml). The average infant consumes 750 ml of milk daily, and the RDA for infants below 12 months of age has been set at 375 mcg RE. Children aged 1 to 3 years are fed solid food containing carotene in addition to milk, and the RDA is increased to 400 RE (300 as retinol, 100 as B-carotene).

The allowance for adult females is 800 RE (4000 IU) or 80 per cent of that for adult males. During pregnancy, the risks of retinol-induced fetal abnormalities are high, particularly in the first trimester. In well nourished women, the recommended daily allowance of 800 mcg RE of vitamin A should be obtained from carotenoid-rich fruits and vegetables in the diet, and self-administered supplements should be avoided, particularly in the first trimester. If supplements are considered necessary in the second and third trimesters to allow for fetal requirements, the recommended daily allowance of 800 RE should not be exceeded, except by physician's prescription.

During lactation, 1300 RE are recommended to provide for the vitamin A excreted in milk. In third world countries where these levels of intake in the diet are not always possible, daily supplements of up to 3000 mcg RE (10,000 IU) have sometimes been advised during pregnancy, to guard against abortion and fetal abnormalities resulting from vitamin A deficiency.

TOXIC DOSES. The regular daily ingestion of supplements exceeding 3000 RE (10,000 IU) by infants and children is not recommended except by direction of a physician, and 7500 RE (25,000 IU) daily is regarded as the maximum safe intake of vitamin A for adults.

Toxicity in adults is reported with daily intakes of more than 15,000 RE (50,000 IU) for long periods. Some authorities have stated that a daily dose of 30,000 RE (100,000 IU) is necessary to induce symptoms of chronic intoxication. The long term toxic daily dose is 10 to 20 times the recommended daily allowance.

Acute intoxication from vitamin A is reported with single doses of 2 million IU in adults and 75,000 IU in infants. These excessive quantities are usually derived from nonprescription commercial vitamin therapies and overdosage with oral retinoids for the treatment of acne. Symptoms of hypervitaminosis A were also observed in infants given periodic mega-supplementation to alleviate chronic vitamin A deficiency, endemic in India and Indonesia. The acute toxic dose is 400 times the recommended daily allowance for adults and 40 times that for infants.

Infants and children are at a greater risk of toxicity from indiscriminate vitamin supplementation. The availability of a popular aqueous emulsion form of vitamin A, which results in much higher blood levels than the older oily preparations, is also a potential hazard. Some cases of hypersensitivity and a genetic predisposition to hypervitaminosis A have been described, and some infants fed normal amounts of baby foods may develop yellow discoloration of the skin because of impaired carotene excretion.

With present day enthusiasm for supplemental vitamins and a common attitude of nonchalance toward possible vitamin overdosage, the recognition of early symptoms and signs of acute and chronic intoxication is important, so that serious and persistent consequences of vitamin abuse may be avoided.

CLINICAL MANIFESTATIONS. *Acute toxicity* has occurred particularly in infants. Symptoms are mainly neurological and include irritability, drowsiness, vomiting, and bulging fontanelle due to raised intracranial pressure. The liver is enlarged and the skin peels after 24 hours. The central nervous system manifestations may mimic cerebral tumor or hemorrhage and lead to unnecessary neurosurgical tests, unless the diagnosis of vitamin A toxicity is suspected and confirmed.

Adults with acute hyper-vitaminosis A complain of headache and dizziness in addition to vomiting. The skin becomes red and swollen and later cracks and peels.

Chronic toxicity affects several systems:

1. General symptoms include fatigue, malaise, abdominal pain, anorexia, nausea, vomiting, low white blood count, and menstrual irregularities;
2. Neurological symptoms are irritability, headache, and increased intracranial pressure, with double vision and papilledema;
3. Skin is dry, itchy, scaly and red, with an eczematoid rash, lips are fissured and bleeding, and the scalp shows alopecia;
4. Bones are painful and show overgrowth, tenderness, epiphyseal closure and resultant growth retardation,
5. Liver and spleen are enlarged, fibrosed and cirrhosed, resulting in jaundice, ascites, and portal hypertension.
6. Blood shows hypercalcemia and anemia.
7. Teratogenic effects. Malformations of the urinary tract, face and head, and central nervous system have been reported following ingestion of 25,000 IU/day

during early pregnancy. Women who delivered a child with spina bifida had significantly elevated serum vitamin A levels.

DIAGNOSIS. The serum retinol level is above 100 mcg/dL (normal 20-60). Radiological studies reveal various bone abnormalities, including hyperostoses of long bones and ribs, metaphyseal cupping, and premature fusion of epiphyses. CT scan or MRI of the head shows small ventricles and changes consistent with pseudotumor cerebri and raised intracranial pressure.

TREATMENT. The increased intracranial pressure gradually resolves after discontinuing vitamin A, and neurosurgical treatment is unnecessary. Rarely, severe refractory cases may require lumbar puncture, steroids, acetazolamide, and mannitol.

Other symptoms gradually improve without treatment.

PROGNOSIS. Full recovery from both acute and chronic hypervitaminosis A is expected, symptoms resolving within one week. Rarely, residual complications include liver disease, bone deformities, optic atrophy, and blindness.

PREVENTION. Megadoses of vitamin A should be avoided, particularly in infants and children and in women during pregnancy. Patients with acne treated with high doses of oral retinoids should be aware of the potential toxicity and presenting symptoms of hypervitaminosis A.

The overzealous use of vitamin therapy as an unproven panacea for various ailments should be discouraged by education and counselling of the general public. Patients with liver disease and chronic renal insufficiency are particularly at risk and may show signs of toxicity with relatively modest doses of vitamin A.

The therapeutic benefit of vitamin A in the prevention and treatment of certain cancers is exciting and promising. Until less toxic retinoid analogs with antitumor activity are developed, the temptation to consume potential overdoses of vitamin A is illadvised. A diet rich in carotenoids would be a safer and probably, a wiser alternative.

VITAMIN D

The importance of vitamin D in human nutrition is its role in the metabolism of calcium and phosphorus. Vitamin D promotes the absorption of these minerals in the intestine and their effects on bone mineralization. When vitamin D is deficient, the mineralization of bone is impaired, resulting in rickets in children and osteomalacea in adults.

Vitamin D is called the "sunshine vitamin" since its production in both plants and animals is dependent on sunlight. It exists in two forms:

1. Vitamin D_2 *(ergocalciferol),* produced by ultraviolet irradiation of the plant sterol, ergosterol; and
2. Vitamin D_3 *(cholecalciferol),* a naturally occurring form in animal tissues, produced by the action of sunlight on 7-dehydrocholesterol in the skin.

The most active form of the vitamin is *dihydroxycholecalciferol,* formed by the hydroxylation of vitamin D_3, first in the liver and then in the kidney.

One international unit (IU) of vitamin D is equivalent to the activity contained in 0.025 mcg of vitamin D3 (cholecalciferol). The recommended daily dietary allowances are expressed as micrograms of cholecalciferol.

SOURCES. Animal foods such as fish, eggs, liver, and butter are natural sources. Unfortified milk is a poor source of vitamin D, and most supplies, including skimmed milk, have cholecalciferol added to provide a concentration of 10 mcg (400 IU) per quart.

Vitamin D formed by the action of sunlight on the skin is generally sufficient for the average white adult. It may be variable in amount and is dependent on a) the length and intensity of sun exposure, 2) atmospheric pollution, and 3) skin color. The sunlight source of vitamin D is limited in dark skinned persons, in infants, and those living in areas where sunlight is inadequate. In these individuals, a dietary source of vitamin D will be necessary to supply the required allowance.

RECOMMENDED ALLOWANCES. The RDA for infants, children, and adolescents is 10 mcg (400 IU), supplied in the diet or as a supplement. For adults aged 25-50 years and over 50 years, the RDA of vitamin D is reduced to 5 mcg (200 IU), since skeletal growth has ceased and the need for calcium is less. During pregnancy and lactation, women require an additional 5 mcg (200 IU).

TOXIC MANIFESTATIONS, The symptoms and signs of hypervitaminosis D are related chiefly to the effects of hypercalcemia and increased excretion of calcium by the kidney. Soft tissues of the body become calcified and bones are demineralized. The arteries and kidneys are damaged, resulting in hypertension and uremia.

Infants with a hypersensitivity to vitamin D fail to thrive and have an unusual elfin-facial appearance, with low-set ears, thick upper lip, and prominent epicanthal eye folds. Hypercalcemia is associated with nausea, vomiting, constipation, increased thirst, and increased urination. Neuromuscular signs include hypotonia, muscle weakness, irritability, and psychomotor retardation. The serum calcium level may be as high as 18 mg/100 ml (normal 10-12).

In adults with normal responsiveness to vitamin D, a daily intake exceeding 50,000 IU is needed to induce toxicity. Those with hypersensitivity to vitamin D, idiopathic hypercalcemia, or diseases such as sarcoidosis and *Mycobacterium* infections develop toxic symptoms with an intake of vitamin D only slightly above normal.

Symptoms of vitamin D intoxication in adults involve the following systems:

- *Muscular* - weakness;
- *Gastrointestinal* - nausea, vomiting, constipation;
- *Urinary* - polyuria, kidney stones;
- *Blood* - elevated calcium level.

TREATMENT. Treatment may require the following: 1) Omission of vitamin D supplements and fortified foods; 2) low calcium diet; and 3) management of severe hypercalcemia with hydration and steroids.

PREVENTION. Vitamin D intake should be limited to the recommended daily allowances, except in certain disease states where supplements may be required and are prescribed by a physician.

Vitamin D is teratogenic in animal models, and women of childbearing potential should be particularly careful to avoid an intake that exceeds the RDA.

VITAMIN E

Vitamin E has been described as a "vitamin in search of a disease." Despite the early disappointments in studies linking vitamin E deficiencies with aging and degenerative disease, claims for the benefits of vitamin E supplements in the prevention and treatment of various ailments now have some scientific validity. The public response to these preliminary findings has involved self-medication with dosages ranging from 100 IU to 1000 IU/daily.

SOURCES. Vitamin E is found in wheat germ, cereals, green leafy vegetables, nuts, legumes, and vegetable oils. The most common synthetic form of the vitamin used in supplements is *dl-a*-tocopheryl acetate supplied in a water solubilized state (1 mg = 1 IU).

FUNCTIONS. Alpha tocopherol, a name derived from the Greek words *tocos* (childbirth) and *phero* (to bear), is a powerful antioxidant. It inhibits the oxidation of unsaturated fatty acids and protects the lipids and integrity of the membranes of tissue cells. Vitamin E is an essential nutrient and plays a fundamental role in maintaining normal muscular, vascular, nervous, and reproductive functions. Symptoms of deficiency include muscle weakness, hemolytic anemia, and neurologic incoordination.

RECOMMENDED ALLOWANCES. The daily dietary allowances of vitamin E are expressed in alpha-tocopherol equivalents (a-TE), as shown in Table 4-1.

1 mg d-a-tocopherol = 1 a-TE = 1.49 IU

The RDA increases from 3 TE in infants under 6 months of age to 10 TE in adolescent and adult males of

15 years and older. Adult females require 8 TE, and 10 and 12 TE during pregnancy and lactation, respectively.

The requirement for vitamin E is related to the intake of polyunsaturated fatty acids (PUFA), as contained in vegetable oils and margarine, fats that are rich in vitamin E. The vitamin E activity in average adult diets in the United States is considered satisfactory.

If the PUFA content of the diet changes or fat absorption is impaired, then the adequacy of the recommended allowances may vary and supplements may be necessary. High fat diets of adults may contain more than 17 mg (25 IU), an intake well above the recommended allowance.

The low-birth-weight infant has a reduced ability to absorb fat, and an oral supplement of 3.3 mg (5 IU) of water soluble a-tocopherol is sometimes recommended or is supplied by a supplemented infant formula. Higher doses (25 IU) used in the prevention of anemia of premature infants have been found toxic and are not advised.

Breast milk contains very high concentrations of vitamin E, and breast-fed term infants attain serum concentrations of vitamin E comparable with those of adults within one week after birth. Supplements of vitamin E are generally unnecessary in breast-fed young infants.

TOXIC MANIFESTATIONS. Vitamin E is generally considered to be relatively innocuous in adults, and supplements of 300 to 800 IU/day have been ingested for months or years without ill effects. In some reports, higher intakes for extended periods have caused muscle weakness, and doses as low as 300 IU/day have induced headaches, fatigue, and gastrointestinal disturbances in a few cases.

Depression of prothrombin levels and hemorrhages may occur as a result of the interference of excess vitamin E with vitamin K activity, particularly in persons with blood clotting disturbances. In normal adults, this risk is small.

Other observed effects of supplemental vitamin E include impaired wound healing, skin rash, low blood sugar, low serum thyroid levels, and an impaired response to iron in children with anemia. High dose vitamin E may increase requirements for vitamins A and D, and some of the toxic effects of hypervitaminoses A and D are prevented with the addition of vitamin E to the diet.

PREVENTION. Vitamin E toxicity is a rare occurrence, except when exceptionally large supplements are ingested over prolonged periods. Adults wishing to take supplements for the possible prevention of cataracts, heart disease, and other degenerative disorders should consult a physician.

VITAMIN K

Vitamin K is essential for the synthesis of prothrombin, a factor important in blood coagulation. Two forms of vitamin K occur naturally, vitamin K_1 in green plants, and vitamin K_2 in bacteria, animals, and man. A synthetic vitamin K_3 (menadione) is used in therapy or as a supplement.

The best dietary sources of vitamin K are green leafy vegetables; fruit, cereals, dairy products, and meat have lesser amounts. The RDA is 1 mcg/kg body weight.

Toxic reactions from vitamin K are rare and never occur with natural dietary sources. Synthetic menadione, however, is potentially toxic, but is not available in over-the-counter vitamin products. Toxicity is therefore restricted to overdose of therapeutic or prophylactic treatment, usually administered intramuscularly by physicians.

Vitamin K3 is given to pregnant women or newborn infants to treat or prevent hemorrhagic disease of the newborn. An increased need for supplementary injections of vitamin K occurs in infants born to mothers who take the anticonvulsant, phenytoin, to prevent epileptic seizures. The phenytoin lowers the blood prothrombin in the mother and newborn infant and predisposes to hemorrhagic disease. Aspirin has a similar effect.

Infants receiving massive doses of vitamin K have developed anemia, jaundice, and kernicterus, an encephalopathy resulting in convulsions, athetoid cerebral palsy, and nerve deafness. Since a safe dose has now been established, this complication of vitamin K injection is rare.

VITAMIN C

Vitamin C was named ascorbic acid because it prevented and cured scurvy. Scurvy is a disease characterized by bleeding into the gums and skin, slow wound healing, and immobility, a pseudoparalysis of painful limbs. Ascorbic acid is synthesized by most animals and plants but not by man. He needs an exogenous source of vitamin C, and this is obtained from fresh, canned, and frozen citrus fruits, tomatoes, potatoes, and leafy vegetables. It is also provided in supplemental tablet form.

Since Linus Pauling advocated vitamin C in megadoses of 3 gm daily for prevention and up to 12 gm daily for the treatment of the common cold, many people have regularly consumed high doses of vitamin C for various ailments, although its benefits remain in doubt. In addition, it is used to improve the absorption of dietary iron, and as an antioxidant and preservative in commercial food products. Vitamin C intake of many persons is higher than the recommended daily allowance and for some, the amount consumed may be potentially toxic.

Although caution in the consumption of megadoses is urged by some authorities, the Joint Expert Committee on Food Additives of the WHO/FAO considers ascorbic acid to be one of the safest constituents of a diet. The acceptable daily intake, defined as the amount of a food additive which may be ingested without any risk of harm, is set at 1050 mg of vitamin C for a 70 kg man. The daily dietary allowances recommended by the revised National Research Council report (1989) are considerably lower than those accepted as nontoxic.

RECOMMENDED ALLOWANCES. A dietary RDA of 60 mg of vitamin C per day is advised for adults of both sexes. Larger amounts are incompletely metabolized, except by regular cigarette smokers who require at least 100 mg of vitamin C per day.

The RDA for infants is based on the amount provided in breast milk. On a body weight basis, the vitamin C requirements of infants and children are higher than that of adults. Infants require 35 mg daily and children up to 11 years of age have an allowance of

45 mg/day. These recommended allowances are considered to meet individual needs and provide a margin of safety.

During pregnancy, plasma vitamin C levels are low, and an additional allowance of 10 mg per day is recommended, particularly in the second and third trimesters. For mothers who breast feed their infants, an additional allowance of 35 mg/day (total 95 mg/day) is recommended, so that a satisfactory level of vitamin C in the breast milk is assured.

TOXIC MANIFESTATIONS. The most common adverse reactions to 1 gm or more megadoses of vitamin C are gastrointestinal disorders such as diarrhea, nausea, and abdominal cramps. Sensitization reactions manifested by urticaria, edema, and skin rashes may also occur.

The greatest concern for vitamin C toxicity is its effects on the kidney and bladder. Ascorbic acid is partially converted into oxalic acid, and its excretion in the urine can increase the risk of stone formation. The passing of kidney stones after taking 2 gm vitamin C daily for only two weeks has been reported. Increased excretion of uric acid in the urine is also noted.

Vitamin C raises the oxygen requirements of cells and tissues. The risk of hypoxia in persons at high altitudes or in those with lung disease may be increased by high dose supplementation of the diet. The ability of ascorbate to enhance iron absorption may not be desirable in men with adequate iron stores, and susceptibility to heart disease may be increased if the intake of vitamin C is excessive.

Large concentrations of ascorbic acid inthe feces interfere with tests for blood in the stools. As little as 55 mg/day excreted in the intestine can result in failure to diagnose gastrointestinal bleeding due to cancer of the colon. When cancer is suspected, patients are advised to avoid all exogenous ascorbic acid for 2-3 days before the test.

High circulating ascorbate levels in the blood can interfere with certain laboratory assays, including the determination of glucose in diabetics, and serum transaminase and bilirubin levels in liver disease. An increase, and less often, a decrease in serum cholesterol has been observed after vitamin C supplements. Interference with the anticoagulant effect of heparin or coumadin drugs has been attributed to the gastrointestinal distress caused by vitamin C megadoses and resultant impaired absorption of the anticoagulant.

The reports of effects of megadoses of vitamin C in the treatment of terminal malignancies are contradictory. Studies have shown reduction of local tumor growth in some patients and stimulation of growth in others. Additional research is warranted.

Prolonged intake of high doses of vitamin C may result in dependency and conditioning, predisposing to rebound scurvy if treatment is suddenly withdrawn. The induction of neonatal scurvy is reported in infants born to mothers who had taken 400 mg/day of ascorbic acid during pregnancy.

PREVENTION. Since many of the claims for beneficial effects of megadoses of vitamin C have not yet been proven, the routine consumption of large supplements to the diet may be premature. However, persons in certain age groups may be at risk for borderline vitamin C deficient states, and supplements larger than those generally recommended may be advisable, particularly in senior citizens who are otherwise healthy.

A recent critical evaluation of the scientific literature dealing with possible side effects of large intakes of ascorbic acid has concluded that the ingestion of up to 10 g vitamin C per day does not constitute a serious health risk for adults. This statement is encouraging for those seeking a panacea for various ailments, but consultation with a physician may be advisable if doses higher than the acceptable safe levels are taken for extended periods.

Persons taking gram doses of vitamin C for long periods of time should reduce intake gradually when discontinuing the supplement.

Women should be alerted to the potential harm to the newborn infant, if excessive doses of vitamin C are taken during pregnancy.

THIAMINE

The primary use of thiamine or vitamin B_1 is in the treatment of beriberi, a deficiency disease characterized by symptoms of nervous and cardiac dysfunction. Berberi occurs in areas where the diet consists of unenriched white rice and white flour. In the United States, alcoholics and patients receiving dialysis for renal disease are those chiefly affected by thiamine deficiency.

Sources of thiamine in the diet include whole-grain or enriched cereals, bread, liver, meats, wheat germ, nuts, legumes, and milk. Large supplementary doses are sometimes prescribed, along with niacin and other vitamins, in the orthomolecular treatment of schizophrenia, autism, and hyperkinetic behavior disorders.

Toxicity is only encountered with parenteral injection therapy. Even at very high doses, oral ingestion of thiamine has not resulted in toxic effects.

Hypersensitivity reactions and anaphylactic shock has occurred with repeated low intravenous injections of thiamine. Doses several hundred times greater than the RDA, administered intravenously, have induced neuromuscular and cardiovascular side effects, including convulsions, weakness, and heart irregularities.

RIBOFLAVIN

Vitamin B2 or riboflavin has a low toxicity, and no case of riboflavin toxicity has been reported in man. The amount absorbed in the intestine is limited by a transport system that becomes saturated.

Riboflavin is rapidly excreted in the urine, giving it a yellow fluorescent color. It may be used in combination with drugs to act as a marker of compliance.

NIACIN

Vitamin B3 or niacin is used in a generic sense for both nicotinic acid and nicotinamide. It is one of the B complex vitamins and is also known as the pellagra-preventive (P-P) factor. The symptoms of pellagra, characterized by the three D's - dementia, dermatitis, and diarrhea, all respond to niacin.

Megadoses of niacin in the range of 3-30 g daily are employed by orthomolecular psychiatrists for the treatment of schizophrenia and other mental disorders. These pharmacological, not nutritional, levels of intake have coincided with reports of niacin toxicity.

TOXIC MANIFESTATIONS. Skin flushing, itching, and vasodilatation occur in all patients receiving nicotinic acid in doses as low as 100 mg orally or 20 mg intravenously. This reaction is accompanied by headache and increased intracranial blood flow. The vasodilation response subsides rapidly even with continued therapy and is not regarded as an untoward side effect.

Higher doses may cause transient gastrointestinal disturbances such as heartburn, nausea, and diarrhea. Other more serious signs of toxicity include high blood sugar in nondiabetics, increased insulin requirements in diabetics, elevated serum uric acid levels and acute gouty arthritis, and duodenal ulcer.

Of greater concern are reports of jaundice and liver damage from chronic niacin therapy, even with doses as low as 750 mg/day. Nicotinamide, which does not cause vasodilatation, is more toxic than nicotinic acid, and its expanding role in orthomolecular therapy carries a higher risk.

Other less frequent side effects of niacin therapy are toxic blindness or optic nerve disease, cardiac fibrillation, skin hyperpigmentation, low thyroid, anxiety, and psychosis. A teratogenic effect has been demonstrated in animal studies.

PREVENTION. The benefits of niacin in lowering serum cholesterol are well established, but its use in treating coronary heart disease patients and neuropsychiatric diseases is controversial. The plethora of published toxic effects must be weighed against the degree of benefit from pharmacological doses of niacin.

Particular caution should be observed in the prescription of high doses of niacin for women of childbearing age and in patients with a history of ulcers, gout, diabetes, and liver disease.

PYRIDOXINE

Vitamin B_6 is a collective term for three naturally occurring pyridine compounds - pyridoxine, pyridoxal, and pyridoxamine. Vitamin B_6 is important in enzyme reactions involved in the metabolism of amino acids, glycogen, and fatty acids. In the brain, pyridoxine participates in the conversion of glutamic acid to gamma-aminobutyric acid (GABA), a function important in neural inhibition. Low levels of GABA in the brain lead to hyperexcitability and convulsions.

Pyridoxine deficency occurs with diabetes, pregnancy, during treatment with certain drugs, especially isoniazid for tuberculosis, and with insufficient intake in the diet. In the early 1950s an outbreak of seizures in more than 300 infants was traced to a pyridoxine deficient formula. The vitamin had been destroyed by the autoclaving process during manufacture of the powder. Infant formulas are now required to be fortified with a supplement of pyridoxine.

A pyridoxine dependency state is reported in occasional infants and young children with seizures resistant to anticonvulsant medications. The addition of pyridoxine in doses of 20 to 200 times the recommended daily allowance is required to control the seizures.

Large doses of pyridoxine in the range of 10 to 100 mg daily have also been used in the treatment of childhood autism, and in adults with carpal-tunnel syndrome, a painful disability involving the median nerve and hand. A pyridoxine deficiency reported in women with emotional problems and related to oral contraceptive use has been relieved by the addition of 25 mg of the vitamin to the diet.

Supplements greater than 25 - 50 mg daily have caused damage to peripheral nerves and are contraindicated unless a true pyridoxine dependency state is established.

TOXIC MANIFESTATIONS. Sensory neuropathy was caused by pyridoxine megadoses of more than 2000 mg daily in one adult and 500 and 200 mg in two additional patients. Improvement followed the withdrawal of the vitamin therapy.

A 34-year-old woman had progressive difficulty in walking after taking pyridoxine in doses of 200 mg daily for a two year period followed by 500 mg daily for one year. Her symptoms began with a sensation of electric shocks down her spine and unsteadiness of gait, especially when she walked in the dark. Later, she complained of a numbness and tingling sensation in her feet, hips, hands, and cheek. She was unable to walk without assistance, and the deep tendon jerks could not be elicited.

The symptoms and signs were suggestive of multiple sclerosis, but the diagnosis of pyridoxine toxicity was considered more likely when improvement followed the withdrawal of the vitamin supplement.

The authors of this report suggested that the marketing of pyridoxine in capsules containing as much as 500 mg and 1000 mg should be discontinued, since the rationale for prescribing megadoses of this magnitude is doubtful.

DRUG INTERACTIONS. Pyridoxine may interact with other drugs and cause undesirable or potentially hazardous effects. Pyridoxine can reverse the therapeutic effect of L-dopa and induce relapse in patients with Parkinsonism. It antagonizes the effects of quinidine in the treatment of tachycardia, penicillamine in the treatment of Wilson's disease, and the antituberculosis agent isoniazid.

The suppression of lactation by pyridoxine supplied in multivitamin preparations is considered a potential hazard by some researchers.

PREVENTION. Doses of pyridoxine larger than 50 - 100 mg daily should be avoided on a regular basis, unless demanded by a vitamin dependency condition.

Nursing mothers should probably limit their intake to the recommended daily allowance of 2.5 mg daily, if continued lactation is desired.

Patients with Parkinsonism, cardiac disease, tuberculosis, and other disorders treated with drugs which interact with pyridoxine should be aware of the potential hazards of vitamin B_6 in supplements and multivitamin preparations.

FOLIC ACID

Folacin is the general term for compounds having nutritional properties and chemical structure similar to those of folic acid. Folacin is present in a wide variety of foods, especially liver, leafy vegetables, fruit, and yeast. Only 25-50 per cent of dietary folacin is nutritionally available.

The 1989 revised daily allowance is set at 200 mcg for the adult male and 180 mcg for the adult female. During pregnancy, the RDA for folate is 400 mcg. The amount contained in the average diet is usually in excess of the RDA.

The requirement for infants is estimated at 3.6 mcg/kg of body weight, or 25 mcg total folacin for infants less than 6 months of age and 35 mcg from 6 months to 1 year of age. Human and cows' milk contains adequate amounts unless the cows' milk is boiled. Boiling destroys heat-labile folacin. Supplements should be given to infants receiving formulas prepared from pasteurized, sterilized, or powdered cows' milk or goats' milk.

The RDAs for children through adolescence range from 50 mcg to the adult value of 200 mcg daily. They are calculated to supply approximately 3 mcg/kg of body weight. During pregnancy, the RDA was set at 800 mcg/day in 1980 and revised to 400 mcg in 1989. For lactating women, a reduction from 500 mcg/day to 280 mcg was considered adequate by 1989 standards.

The Center for Disease Control in Atlanta has recently recommended that all women of childbearing age, and particularly those who have given birth to an infant with spina bifida, anencephaly, cleft palate or cleft lip, should take a daily supplement of 0.4 mg of folic acid in addition to that supplied in the diet. Folic acid in a 4 mg daily dosage or multivitamins has been found to decrease the incidence of recurrence of neural tube defects in subsequent planned pregnancies.

Low maternal serum folate levels have been associated with a significantly greater incidence of birth defects in infants whose mothers were taking anticonvulsant medication for epilepsy. When folic acid supplements (2.5-5 mg/day) were given, all infants were born alive and none had birth defects. Unfortunately, folic acid may antagonize the effectiveness of the anticonvulsant drug and result in an exacerbation of the epilepsy.

TOXIC REACTIONS. In addition to the effect on epilepsy by interreaction with anticonvulsant drugs, folic acid may interfere with the treatment of pernicious anemia. In doses greater than 1 mg/day, folic acid corrects the anemia of vitamin B_{12} deficiency but does not prevent neurological complications. Excessive folate supplementation without added vitamin B_{12} may result in irreversible spinal nerve degeneration, optic atrophy and other neurological damage. Prophylactic vitamin supplements should always include vitamin B_{12} along with folic acid.

Hypersensitivity reactions to folic acid have been reported folowing repeated daily doses as small as 3 mg orally in adults and in an infant whose mother received injections of folic acid during pregnancy. Fever, urticaria, and erythema of the skin occurred with small oral supplements, whereas the reaction was anaphylactoid and life-threatening following injections of higher doses.

In doses of 20 mg daily, folic acid supplements have been associated with gastrointestinal upset, sleep disturbances, and mental symptoms, including anxiety, impaired concentration, irritability, and hyper-excitability.

PREVENTION. Folic acid supplements not exceeding 15 mg/day are believed to be safe in normal subjects. During pregnancy, the supplement should not exceed 0.4 mg/day, or 4 mg daily in high risk mothers. In patients with epilepsy, folic acid should be taken only after consultation with the neurologist.

VITAMIN PUBLIC AWARENESS

With the recent surge of interest in vitamin supplements to improve cognitive functioning of children and delay aging and degenerative disorders of adults, it is especially important to emphasize the potentially harmful effects of inappropriate administration of vitamins.

In a recent questionnaire study in England involving the parents of 120 children attending child health clinics, the responses showed that almost half the parents were unaware that overdosage of vitamins was potentially harmful, and 22 percent of the children were given the wrong dose. Vitamins were administered without the advice of a physician or nurse in 90 percent of the children in this study.

Public awareness of the benefits and potential hazards of vitamin supplements should be expanded by improvements in health professional supervision. The daily dietary allowances of vitamins (RDAs) recommended by the US National Research Council are shown in the following Table 4-1. Doses exceeding these levels over extended periods should be taken cautiously and usually with the approval of a physician.

TABLE 4-1. Recommended Daily Dietary Allowances of Vitamins (RDAs), National Research Council, 1989.

Vitamin	*Adult Males*	*Adult Females*	*Pregnant Females*
Vitamin A	1000 RE	800 RE	800 RE
Vitamin D	10-5 mcg	10-5 mcg	10 mcg
Vitamin E	10 mg	8 mg	10 mg
Vitamin C	60 mg	60 mg	70 mg
Thiamin	1.5 mg	1.1 mg	1.5 mg
Riboflavin	1.7 mg	1.3 mg	1.6 mg
Niacin	19 mg	15 mg	17 mg
Vitamin B_6	2.0 mg	1.6 mg	2.2 mg
Folic Acid	200 mcg	180 mcg	400 mcg

See text and reference for further details.

Gaby SK, Bendich A, Singh VN, Machlin LJ. Vitamin Intake and Health. A Scientific Review. New York, M Dekker, 1991.

Ko MLB, Ramsell N, Wilson JA. What do parents know about vitamins? Arch Dis Child 67: 1080, 1992.

Machlin LJ (ed). Handbook of Vitamins, 2nd ed. New York, Marcel Dekker, 1991.

Miller DR, Hayes KC. Vitamin excess and toxicity. In: Hathcock JN. (ed). Nutritional Toxicology vol 1. New York, Academic Press, 1982.

Millichap JG. Nutrition, Diet, and Your Child's Behavior. Facts and Current Issues. Springfield,Illinois, Charles Thomas,1986.

Noji EK, Kelen GR. Manual of Toxicological Emergencies. Chicago, Year Book Med Publishers, 1989.

CHAPTER 5

FOOD ADDITIVE TOXICITY

"Aspartame: Some Bitter with the Sweet?"
Science 5:14, 1984.

Food additives such as salt, sugar, and spices have been used for hundreds of years, but the change from an agricultural to an industrial society created the need for highly processed convenience products and a wider variety of food stabilizers, flavorings, colors, and preservatives. In the United States, distribution systems to supply the cities with food were established at the turn of the century, but conditions were often unsanitary and dangerous.

According to Robert Dean of the Food and Nutrition Service, United States Department of Agriculture, in the early 1900s "it was relatively common for floor sweepings to be added to pepper, ash leaves to tea, copper and lead salts to cheese and candy, copper salts to pickles and peas, prussic acid to wine, alum to bread, acorns to coffee, and brick dust to cocoa. Fruit jams or jellies were made with water, dextrose, grass seed, and color."

The publication of the book, *The Jungle,* by Upton Sinclair in 1906, an expose of the Chicago meat-packing industry, prompted an investigation by President Roosevelt and the Federal Government that culminated in the Pure-Food Legislation.

FEDERAL FOOD LEGISLATION

The Federal Food and Drug Act of 1906, often referred to as the "Pure Food Law," prohibited the manufacture and shipment of adulterated or misbranded foods and drugs. A "poison squad" of young men who were paid to consume manufactured products was used to establish the safety of chemicals commonly used in foods. Of seven synthetic color additives permitted in those times, only two are presently approved.

With the passage into law of the **Food, Drug, and Cosmetic Act** (FD&C) of 1938, the certification of individual lots of 15 synthetic colors became mandatory, and standards of identity for individual food products were established.

In 1947, the **Federal Insecticide, Fungicide and Rodenticide Act** regulated the composition of insecticides, and required that these so-called economic poisons be registered, and have added color to prevent confusion with flour, sugar, salt, or other edibles. The law stipulated that the container should have the word "poison" in red, a skull and crossbones, and an antidote to the poison prominently displayed.

The FD&C Act was amended in 1954 to establish tolerances for the amounts of economic poisons allowed to remain in or on fruits, vegetables, and agricultural produce. This law, commonly known as the **Miller Amendment**, is a function of the Environmental Protection Agency (EPA). While the EPA is responsible for establishing tolerances for pesticides, the FDA monitors and assures compliance with the tolerances for agricultural commodities.

In establishing tolerances, the EPA includes meat, fat, milk, and animal feeds, as well as fruits and vegetables for human consumption. An amendment to the FD&C Act in 1960 allowed foods treated with pesticides to be supplied to consumers without their presence listed on the label.

In 1958, a **Food Additives Amendment** was added to the FD&C Act designed "*to prohibit the use in foods of additives which have not been adequately tested to establish their safety.*"

FOOD ADDITIVE DEFINITION. As defined by law, "*any substance the intended use of which results or may reasonably be expected to result, directly or indirectly, in its becoming a component or otherwise affecting the characteristics of any food (including any substance intended for use in producing, manufacturing, packing, processing, preparing, treating, packaging, transporting or holding food; and including any source of radiation intended for any such use), if such substance is not generally recognized among experts......to be safe under the conditions of its intended use.....*"

The term **"Generally Recognized As Safe" (GRAS)** was used by industry and government for lists of substances which were considered safe for use in food.

Food additives causing cancer in animals or humans were prohibited at any level of tolerance by the **Delaney Amendment** to the FD&C Act. This amendment resulted in controversy, its proponents holding it essential to protect the health of consumers, while its detractors felt it too restrictive . Theoretically, this *zero-risk mandate* is the optimal method of ensuring the safety of food supplies, but realistically, a balance of risks and benefits were considered necessary in food additive regulations.

The efforts of the FDA to limit quantities of colors used in foods were opposed in the courts, and this prompted the passage of the **Color Additive Amendments** of 1960. The burden of testing and proof of safety of color additives was shifted to industry, and the FDA was responsible for proscribing tolerance limitations, exemptions from certification, and labeling requirements.

The Poultry Products Act of 1957 and the **Wholesome Poultry Products Act** of 1968 called for inspection of poultry and a statement of ingredients, including artificial flavors, colors, or preservatives, on the label. **The Fair Packaging and Labelling Act** of 1966 was designed to inform consumers of the composition of packaged goods. Nutritional labeling of food products and nutrient requirements for infant formulas were regulated in 1973 and 1980, repectively.

A major change in regulation of the meat packing industry occurred with the passage of the

Wholesome Meat Act of 1967. A carcass or meat product was adulterated if it contained any added substance injurious to health or any substance administered to the live animal which was poisonous or deleterious to humans. Meat subjected to radiation was also included in the definition of adulterated food.

The Toxic Substances Control Act of 1976 required testing for carcinogenesis, mutagenesis, teratogenesis, and behavioral disorders caused by chemicals, but food additives were excluded from this legislation.

The regulation of food additives is a constant topic of debate. The United States food supply is among the safest in the world, but surveys have indicated that the American public does not trust government regulation of food additives to completely protect the consumer from potential adverse effects. The carcinogenic effects of certain chemicals over time is a particular concern of many.

A completely risk free food supply cannot be guaranteed, but the highly sophisticated testing techniques presently available have made risk assessment more accurate. Scientists who evaluate the safety of additives use laboratory animals, not the food-testing human volunteer squads as formerly employed. Animals are fed huge doses of the substance to be tested, so that a wide margin of safety is intended for increased consumer protection.

Food Additive Research. The future of food additive research is directed toward the mechanisms of chemical carcinogenesis and the correlation of data obtained from animals with the risk of toxicity to humans. The behavioral effects of additives have assumed importance since preservatives and dyes were believed to cause hyperactivity in children. Elimination diets and challenge studies were found necessary to define the small but significant role of food additives in the behavioral and learning disorders of young children.

Food additives certified as GRAS include preservatives, processing agents, flavorings, and colorings.

FOOD PRESERVATIVES

Nitrites, antioxidants, and sulfites are the chief preservative additives used to prevent changes in color, flavor and texture when food is exposed to air.

NITRITES. Nitrites are used to cure bacon and other pork products. They protect the consumer from botulism. Unfortunately, nitrites convert to nitrosamines by combining with amides and amines in the body. Nitrosamines are among the most potent carcinogens.

In response to this risk of cancer from eating bacon and other nitrite containing pork products, the FDA has lowered the acceptable level of nitrites to the minimum required to prevent botulism. Nitrosamine formation in nitrite-cured meats is inhibited by the addition of an antioxidant, ascorbate or alpha-tocopherol.

ANTIOXIDANTS. These also have been linked to cancer in laboratory animals. BHA (butylated hydroxyanisole) and BHT (butylated hydroxytoluene) are the antioxidants most widely used. Their purpose is to prevent lipid-containing baking mixes, instant potatoes, cereals, and other products from turning rancid on exposure to air and oxygen.

In 1983, a study showed that rats fed BHA for two years developed papilloma tumors of the forestomach. Further investigations of this carcinogenic effect have demonstrated the induction of tumors in the stomach and precancerous lesions in the esophagus of other animals after shorter periods of exposure to BHA.

In combination with nitrite, under acidic conditions simulating the gastric contents, BHA resulted in the formation of highly mutagenic products. Since many foods contain nitrite or nitrate, which is converted into nitrite by bacteria in the mouth, the combination of BHA as a preservative could have serious toxicological implications.

BHT fed rats developed lung and liver tumors but not stomach tumors. As with BHA, BHT may interact with known carcinogens and mutagens, or DNA-damaging chemicals. However, the effects are sometimes inconclusive and contradictory.

In addition to the carcinogenic question, BHT has also caused internal and external hemorrhaging in many different species of animals, severe enough to cause death. The mechanism of the bleeding tendency is a lowering of prothrombin levels; it may be prevented by the administration of vitamin K. The mechanism is similar to that of vitamin E-induced hemorrhage, and is related to a reduction in vitamin K-dependent clotting factors.

As a result of these disturbing findings, Japan has banned BHA as a preservative in foods. The United

States has determined that further research is needed before these antioxidants are removed from the GRAS list of acceptable certified food additives. It is not surprising that consumers are unconvinced of the safety of additives and some favor their elimination from foods.

SULFITES. The term "sulfiting agents" includes sulfur dioxide, sodium sulfite, sodium metabisulfite, sodium bisulfite, potassium metabisulfite, and potassium bisulfite. Sulfites inhibit bacteria and prevent undesirable browning in fresh fruits and vegetables. They are also used as preservatives in dried fruits and dehydrated potatoes and in wines.

Until 1986, sulfites were classified as GRAS. As a result of deaths from hypersensitivity reactions to sulfites used in restaurant salad bars, the FDA withdrew the GRAS status of sulfites as preservatives of fruits and vegetables. Occurring mostly in patients with asthma, the reactions were characterized by angioedema, bronchospasm, urticaria, flushing, tachycardia, low blood pressure, and in some cases, respiratory arrest.

One young adult patient, a wine salesman who suffered from asthma, developed a sensitivity to sulfites in the wine. After several near fatal reactions and visits to hospital emergency rooms, he decided to resign his job. He has continued to react to sulfites encountered in salads and some undetermined sources. Fortunately, he has married a nurse he met at the hospital, who, along with close friends, is often called to render life-saving resuscitation.

However careful, patients sometimes unwittingly eat foods containing sulfites. Sulfites are still allowed on grapes as a fungicide agent, but the EPA is reviewing the safety of this permit. Products containing more than 10 ppm must have the term "sulfiting agents" declared on the label.

FOOD FLAVORINGS

Approximately 800 synthetic flavoring substances and adjuvants are listed by the FDA as safe for use in foods with limitations. Monosodium glutamate and artificial sweeteners are the most controversial items in this group of food additives.

MONOSODIUM GLUTAMATE. The Chinese Restaurant Syndrome has been linked to the frequent use of monosodium glutamate (MSG) in chinese food. Consumers reported flushing, tingling, dizziness, and headache. Patients with migraine had exacerbations of their symptoms.

CYCLAMATES. Cyclamates largely superseded saccharin as a non-nutrative sweetener in the late 1950s and 1960s. A mixture of cyclamate and saccharin fed to mice and rats was found to cause bladder tumors and, in 1968, the FDA banned cyclamate as a sweetener for human consumption. Subsequent studies have suggested that cyclamate may not be a true carcinogen, but rather a promoter or cocarcinogen.

SACCHARIN. After 70 years of use, the FDA enforced the Delaney Clause and banned saccharin because of bladder tumors and a carcinogenic effect similar to that discovered with cyclamates in rats. Congress reacted by placing a moratorium on the ban.

The National Cancer Institute study of artificial sweeteners and bladder cancer in over 9000 persons failed to demonstrate a significant risk from saccharin for the general population, but pointed to subgroups, particularly non-smoking white females, who may be at increased risk. The ban on saccharin has been contested but the controversy continues.

ASPARTAME. Marketed under the trade name of *NutraSweet,* aspartame appears to be free from risks of carcinogenicity, but the potential hazards of its metabolites as a cause of brain dysfunction have resulted in controversy and much adverse publicity.

The FDA approved aspartame in July 1981 as a tabletop sugar substitute and additive in dry foods and beverage bases, such as cold breakfast cereals, chewing gums, instant coffee and tea, pudding and pie filling mixes, and nondairy whipped toppings. In 1983, aspartame was also approved for inclusion in soft drinks such as diet sodas. Whereas one teaspoonful of sugar contains 16 calories, a tabletop sweetener with NutraSweet contains only two calories for the same amount of sweetness.

Effect on Brain Chemistry. Aspartame is broken down in the body to form methanol, aspartic acid, and phenylalanine. Phenylalanine is especially toxic to patients with phenylketonuria (PKU).

Studies in animals have shown that aspartame almost doubles brain phenylalanine levels. and this increase is fourfold if aspartame is consumed along with carbohydrates. The normal increases in brain serotonin, a neurotransmitter substance, produced by a carbohydrate meal, are blocked by aspartame.

All NutraSweet products are labelled with an FDA warning to parents of children with PKU that the product contains phenylalanine. The ingestion of aspartame by phenylketonurics could reverse the beneficial effects of the low-phenylalanine diet prescribed to prevent mental retardation.

Symptoms of Aspartame Toxicity. In 1984, the Center for Disease Control (CDC) in Atlanta, at the invitation of the FDA, investigated complaints of headache, dizziness, alterations of mood and other neurological and behavioral symptoms associated with the consumption of aspartame. The CDC concluded that, "Although it may be that certain individuals have an unusual sensitivity to the product (aspartame), these data do not provide evidence for the existence of serious, widespread, adverse health consequences attendant to the use of aspartame."

Despite the FDA decision to clear aspartame for general consumption, excepting phenylketonuric children, many scientists expressed caution with its use in patients with migraine and epilepsy, and especially in children with neuropsychiatric problems. In recent years, several studies have demonstrated that headaches may be exacerbated in patients suffering from migraine. Children with petit mal epilepsy have an increased frequency of electroencephalographic seizure discharges when aspartame-containing drinks are permitted.

Clearly, the questions regarding safety of aspartame have not been answered satisfactorily, and the FDA clearance for general consumption may be premature. Further research independent of the manufacturer and supported by governmental funds should be continued.

COLOR ADDITIVES

ARTIFICIAL COLORS. Toxic reactions linked to color additives have included hyperkinetic behavior in children and allergic reactions, particularly in persons who are also sensitive to aspirin.

Color additives permitted in foods include Red Dye No. 3 (Erythrosine), Red 40, Citrus Red 2, Yellow No. 5 (Tartrazine), Yellow No. 6, Green No. 3, and Blue Nos 1 and 2. Azo dyes such as tartrazine have provoked allergic reactions, and Red No. 3 is a suspected carcinogen.

Several color additives, including Red No. 1, Red No. 4, No. 2, Violet No. 1, Green No. 1, carbon black, and graphite, were banned from the list of GRAS substances for use in foods between 1960 and 1977 because of suspected carcinogenicity. The dyes, Red Nos. 8, 9, 19, and 37, and Orange No. 17 are also known carcinogens. Most are currently listed for use in cosmetics and drugs.

NATURAL COLORS. The FDA lists natural substances that are GRAS as flavoring agents and color additives that are exempt from certification. The list of natural colors includes beets, caramel, carotene, carrot oil, cochineal extract or carmine, grape color extract, and turmeric. Carotene is also supplied synthetically. Recently, the FDA has raised questions about the precise chemical composition of various forms of caramel used as color additives.

In the face of increasing questions about composition and toxicology raised by regulators, and a relative lack of commercial interest in natural compared to synthetic products, the future development of natural additives is bleak. The exceptions are colors that are also nutrients, such as riboflavin, carotene, and related substances; caramel, used in large quantities: and cochineal extract, with a specific application. Many others may not receive sufficient interest and support to allow the expense of tests of safety.

FOOD ADDITIVES AND HYPERKINESIS

In the 1970s Feingold popularized a theory that certain food additives were the cause of hyperactivity and other behavioral disorders in children. Treatment with a diet that eliminated salicylates, artificial colors, and the preservatives BHT and BHA was reportedly successful.

Scientific panels, established to study the efficacy of the diet and sponsored by the FDA, criticized the treatment for lack of controls and statistical validity. Numerous studies of the effects of food additives on behavior followed, including additive-containing challenges. Small subgroups of younger children were found to react adversely to color additives in short term trials, but the overwhelming benefits claimed by Dr. Feingold were not substantiated.

The proof of food additive toxicity and causal relation to hyperactive behavior is difficult to determine. Questionnaires completed by parents, teachers, and psychologists may be biased, for or against, and may not address behavioral symptoms susceptible to the additive or elimination therapy.

Interest in the Feingold hypothesis and dietary treatment of hyperactive behavior has waned in the United States but waxes in Europe, where research continues on the use of elimination and hypoallergenic diets for the treatment of a variety of childhood neurobehavioral disorders.

FUTURE OF FOOD ADDITIVE SAFETY

The future of food additive research should emphasize the mechanisms of chemical carcinogenesis, the most serious potential hazard attending their use. Methods employed in correlating animal data with risks to the consumer must be more reliable. The health of the individual should take precedence over the manufacturer's interests and commercial gain.

Adverse effects of food additives on behavior, learning, neuropsychiatric disorders, and reproduction and early fetal development have assumed importance in addition to carcinogenic effects. These hazards will need to be addressed in testing new food additives.

Various points of view are expressed in a compilation of more than 250 recent articles published in the Orynx Science Bibliographies, 1988. In some accounts, the FDA is criticized for excessive regulation and in others, for too little. Those opposed to the Delaney Clause and its "zero risk" approach to food additives find it too limiting, and a risk/benefit method of evaluation is proposed as an alternative.

Consumer magazine articles show food safety to be a high priority in public opinion polls. A fear of chemicals and artificial ingredients, and a lack of confidence in government research are stressed. A greater reliance on natural additives would be preferred by many, but lack of detailed information on the composition of natural colors is a concern of regulators. "Naturalness" per se offers no assurance of safety, and toxicological data similar to those required for artificial additives may be necessary in certain circumstances.

The food industry and FDA officials feel that the American public have an exaggerated fear of chemicals in their food. In their opinion, the greatest foodborne danger comes from microbiological contamination, not food additives.

In the general population, the benefits of food additives probably outweigh the risks, but for certain individuals, particularly those with allergic hypersensitivity disorders, some additives carry a real and serious hazard. A problem in dealing with food additive sensitivity is the difficulty in determining when certain additives, particularly sulfites, have been added to processed food or fruit.

Labelling of additives in produce, both processed and fresh, needs to be clear and prominent, with warnings to asthmatics and other susceptible consumers of potential dangers. Health magazine editors have addressed the subject, but the role of government and industry in the education of the public regarding the pros and cons of food additives needs to be expanded. If a risk assessment approach to food additive regulation is to be accepted, the consumer must be better informed of risks and benefits and alternative methods of ensuring safety of the food supply.

Food irradiation is one alternative technique for preserving and improving the safety of food. Legally, it is considered a food additive. At present, the main barrier to a wider use of irradiated foods is lack of consumer acceptance. The evolving regulation and public education concerning food irradiation is discussed in the following chapter.

Berdick M. Safety of food colors. In: HathcockJN (ed) Nutritional Toxicology vol 1, New York, Academic Press, 1982.

Dean RW. Food additives. Their regulatory status. Their use by the food industry. In: Lewis RJSr. Food Additives Handbook. New York, Van Nostrand, 1989.

Feingold BF. Why Your Child is Hyperactive. New York, Random House, 1975.

Food Irradiation. Geneva. World Health Organization, 1988.

Harley JP, Matthews CG, Eichman P. Synthetic food colors and hyperactivity in children: Double-blind challenge experiment. Pediatrics 62: 975, 1978.

Hudson BJF. Food Antioxidants. London, Elsevier Science Publishers, 1990.

Huls ME. Food additives and their impact on health. In: Tyckoson DA (ed). Oryx Science Bibliographies vol 12. Oryx Press, 1988.

Millichap JG. Nutrition, Diet, and Your Child's Behavior. Springfield, Illinois, Charles C Thomas, 1986.

CHAPTER 6

FOOD IRRADIATION

The use of ionizing radiation for food processing is considered a food additive. Irradiation has the same objective as other food processing methods, which include chemical treatment, drying, heat, freezing, and fermentation. The aim is to reduce spoilage and deterioration and to control the growth of microbes causing foodborne diseases.

The spoilage of food, especially in developing countries, is an enormous world-wide problem, sometimes amounting to 50 percent. Raw foods of animal origin are often contaminated by bacteria which can result in foodborne illnesses. Meat and meat products are prone to infestation with trichinosis and toxoplasmosis, both causing serious disease in man. The exposure of food to ionizing radiation can reduce infestation by insects and contamination by organisms and will retard the spoilage of food.

Public acceptance of food irradiation has been slow because of fears of nuclear war and nuclear accidents, such as Three Mile Island in the USA and Chernobyl in Russia. Furthermore, the safety of irradiated food has been questioned. Does irradiation make food radioactive? Are there long-term ill-effects from eating irradiated foods? Could "radiolytic products," or compounds formed in food processed by irradiation, be injurious to our health?

The World Health Organization in collaboration with the Food and Agriculture Organization of the United Nations is concerned with the provision of safe and nutritious food supplies, and especially with the pressing problem of impending starvation in some third world countries. The acceptance and more general use of food irradiation would simplify the task of delivery of processed and stored food to populations in need. The WHO, with contributions from a number of experts, has prepared a publication attempting to dispel the fears of the public and encouraging the more general use of irradiation in food preservation.

FOOD IRRADIATION PROCESS

The sources of ionizing radiation used in the process of food irradiation are man-made radionuclides and machines. Radionuclides are radioactive materials that give off ionizing gamma-rays as they decay. The FDA allows gamma rays from sealed units of the radionuclides, cobalt-60 or cesium-137, to be used in the process.

The machines employed in the process are electron accelerators and X-ray generators. Electrons generated by a machine not to exceed 10 million electron volts, and X-rays not to exceed 5 million electron volts are permitted as sources of ionizing radiation for the processs of food irradiation.

Radiation Dose. The radiation dose or quantity of radiation energy absorbed by the food is measured in *grays* (Gy). The maximum dose recommended by the WHO for use in food irradiation is 10,000 grays (10 kGy).

A specific dose has to be used for each different kind of food. If the dose is too low, the intended effect will not be achieved; if too high, the food product may be damaged.

•Low doses (0.05-1.0 kGy) are used to inhibit sprouting of potatoes; for disenfestation of cereals, fruit, and pork; and to delay ripening of fresh fruits and vegetables.

•Medium doses (1-10 kGy) extend shelf life of fish and strawberries; and eliminate spoilage and bacteria from fish, poultry, and meat.

•High doses (10-50 kGy) are needed for sterilization of hospital diets and are not yet endorsed by the WHO.

The radiation dose commonly used in food processing ranges from 50 Gy to 10 kGy and varies according to the type of food and the effect desired. At these levels ionizing radiation is considered to be safe but with certain limitations.

UNWANTED EFFECTS OF FOOD IRRADIATION

•**Undesirable flavor.** No satisfactory method has been found to prevent an off-flavor in irradiated dairy products and fresh meats. Lean cuts are affected more than meat with a high fat content. The dose required to control *Trichinella* infestation of pork is small and less likely to cause an off-flavor.

•**Discoloration.** Relatively low radiation doses can cause a brown discoloration of meat that is exposed to air.

•**Softening.** The break down of cell membranes results in softening of some fruits. The effect is noticeable some hours or even days after irradiation. Soups and gravies containing starch become thinner and less viscous.

•**Loss of nutrients.** Vitamins A, B_1, E, and K may be destroyed, while vitamin D, riboflavin, and niacin are more resistant to irradiation. The effect on vitamin C is variable, and that on folic acid is undetermined. The cumulative loss of vitamins through processing and cooking could make supplements to the diet mandatory.

•**Bacterial spore resistance.** Botulism, a serious foodborne disease, may not be prevented by irradiation doses sufficient to destroy salmonella microorganisms.

•**Incomplete destruction of bacteria.** Temperature and moisture content of food are correlated directly with the sensitivity of organisms to irradiation. Microorganisms are less sensitive to radiation when contained in cold, dry food than when incorporated in a warm, watery suspension. A proportion of the bacteria is not killed but may be injured. This can pose a public health problem if the irradiated food is not stored in the frozen state.

•**Chromosomal changes.** Malnourished children fed freshly irradiated wheat reportedly showed more chromosomal abnormalities than those fed irradiated wheat after prolonged storage.

Laboratory and other population studies failed to confirm this disturbing report, and the significance of the findings is unclear.

• **Radiolytic effects.** Chemical changes in food induced by irradiation are dose dependent. They occur with moderate to high doses. The changes are not unique to irradiated foods, and the chemicals formed cannot be used to identify foods that have been irradiated.

AVAILABILITY OF IRRADIATED FOODS

Food irradiation has been approved in 33 countries for 30 food products. In the United States, the list is relatively long, and includes wheat, flour, potatoes, spices, pork, fresh foods, and enzyme preparations, available to the general public. In the United Kingdom, availability is restricted to hospital patients who require a sterilized diet as an essential part of their treatment.

The need for processed foods is greater in the United States, where supplies are transported over great distances, than in countries like England, where the consumer is located closer to the site of food production. Despite the practical advantages of the irradiation process, the demand for a commercial market is not large. A wider public understanding of the details of the process might increase consumer acceptance, but the fear of irradiation will remain as a marketing deterrent and difficult barrier to overcome.

IDENTIFYING IRRADIATED FOODS

The product carries a label that states "Treated with radiation" or "Treated by irradiation." All retail packages of foods that are irradiated are required to be marked with the logo, as shown in Fig. 6-1.

All meat and poultry products that contain irradiated pork show this symbol and label, but the FDA does not require foods that include irradiated ingredients to have this disclosure on the package. We may be eating irradiated food and not know it!

Foods that have been irradiated once must not be treated again. If an irradiated food is shipped to another manufacturer for further processing, it must contain the statement, "Treated with radiation-do not irradiate again."

Labelling practices vary from country to country, but the symbol is gaining acceptance as a trademark for food processed with ionizing radiation.

DANGERS OF RADIOACTIVITY IN FOOD

The adverse effects of ionizing radiation on the developing nervous system are well known. Radioactive iodine from nuclear power plants or nuclear explosions in the atmosphere is more dangerous than food contamination. Strontium-90 is present in food, particularly milk and dairy products, as a result of nuclear testing, an example of environmental-nutritional pollution. Strontium-90 has a long half-life, it accumulates in bone, and it may cause disease of the bone-marrow and blood.

Exposure of the body to ionizing radiation produces free radicals that are involved in chemical changes, resulting in carcinogenic, mutagenic, and teratogenic effects. Intensive doses cause radiation sickness. The effects of irradiation exposure through food contamination would vary with the half-life of the isotope. If short half-life radionuclides are employed in food irradiation, the risk is small, whereas products contaminated with longer half-life radionuclides would be hazardous.

The World Health Organization assures us that food irradiated under approved conditions does not become radioactive, and that the treatment does not alter the food in any way that could be harmful to people. Public acceptance of this reassuring statement will be hampered by the fears of accidental exposure to unapproved excessive doses of irradiation, and a lack of information regarding regulatory legislation and governmental controls.

Dean RW. Food additives. In: Food Additives Handbook. New York, Van Nostrand, 1989.

Food Irradiation. Geneva, World Health Organization, 1988.

Norton S. Effects of food chemicals on behavior of experimental animals. In: Hathcock JN (ed). Nutritional Toxicology, vol 1. New York, Academic Press, 1982.

Radionuclides in Foods. Washington, DC, National Academy of Sciences, 1973.

Urbain WM. Food Irradiation. New York, Academic Press, 1986.

Fig. 6-1. Logo for food product treated with irradiation.
Reproduced from "Food Irradiation, 1988," with permission from World Health Organization, Geneva.

CHAPTER 7

ENVIRONMENTAL POISONS

Foods may be contaminated by a wide variety of chemicals that are introduced into the environment by man, either intentionally or by accident. Environmental contaminants that can affect our food supply include PCBs (polychlorinated biphenyls), PBBs (polybrominated biphenyls), aflatoxins, nitrites, nitrates, nitroso compounds, DDT, dioxin, and metals such as mercury and lead.

DDT and other pesticides, including dioxin, dieldrin and chlordane, have been banned since 1972. PCBs have not been produced since 1976. Despite the fact that these and other chemicals are no longer made, dangerous concentrations persist in the water of inland lakes. From the sediment at the bottom of harbors where they were dumped years ago, hazardous waste residues pollute the water and are eaten by microscopic organisms. From fish the pesticides are passed on to birds and humans, causing a wide range of adverse effects.

A recent study conducted by the Environmental Protection Agency has shown environmental pollutants, PCB, Dioxin, Mercury, and DDT breakdown products, in samples of Lake Michigan water taken from various sites. Historically, environmental toxicology studies in the Great Lakes basin began in the 1950s when declines in lake trout and in 14 species of wildlife were correlated with DDT and PCB contamination of the lake water.

Problems caused by these pollutants in Lake Michigan include the following:

•Fish, especially large trout, are deemed unsafe to eat by the four states bordering Lake Michigan--Illinois, Indiana, Wisconsin and Michigan.

•Fish and wildlife populations are falling.

•Pollutants have reduced the numbers of plankton in the lake, affecting the food chain base.

Studies of this type should help regulators of toxic wastes to pinpoint the chief sources and offenders and find programs to clean up the PCBs and other pollutants in our environment.

PCB

Food becomes contaminated with PCBs mainly via freshwater fish, exposed by leakage into rivers and inland lakes. Spillage on animal feeds will subsequently contaminate animal food products. The biological magnification of the hazard is most apt to occur in aquatic food chains; these contain more links than terrestial food chains. Man is the final consumer in both types of food chains, and he is exposed to the greatest concentrations of any environmental poison.

While regulatory control measures have substantially reduced the PCB contamination of animal feeds and food products, those subgroups of the population who regularly consume fish caught in lakes and streams are still at risk. Surveys and analyses of fish from the Hudson river in New York State and from Lake Michigan showed significant levels of contamination with PCBs in excess of 5 ppm.

Most species of fish were affected, and residue levels were proportional to the age and size of the fish. Trout and salmon had the highest levels of contamination, and whitefish had the lowest PCB residues.

Studies designed to assess the health hazard of PCB exposure from Lake Michigan fish showed a positive correlation between the quantity of fish consumed and the concentration of PCB in blood and breast milk of participants. Those eating higher amounts of fish had significantly higher blood levels of PCB. In other studies, PCBs were reported in samples of malignant breast tissue. Children born to women who routinely consumed Lake Michigan sportfish displayed poorer short-term memory function on both verbal and quantitative tests in a dose-dependent fashion.

Clinical Manifestations of PCB Poisoning. The symptoms attributed to PCB human exposure include acne, skin pigmentation, eye discharge, visual impairment, weakness, numbness, headaches, and liver dysfunction. Infants born to mothers exposed to PCB were pigmented, and the skin discoloration disappeared as the child became older. The adults experienced a slow improvement in the symptoms and eventual recovery. These observations were recorded in Japanese families exposed to PCB in 1968, when a heat exchanger leaked PCB into rice oil (Yusho).

Later reports suggested that the rice oil may have contained an additional polychlorinated contaminant that could have contributed to the symptoms.

PBB

The similarities in trade names for a dairy feed supplement, *NutriMaster*, and an industrial flame retardant, *FireMaster* BP-6, led to a mixup in bags and the accidental PBB poisoning of several dairy herds, hogs, and poultry in Michigan in 1973. FireMaster, containing the polybrominated biphenyls, PBBs, was used in the manufacture of typewriters, radios, and small parts for TV and electrical installations. Both FireMaster and NutriMaster were made by the same company.

The cattle and swine refused to eat, lost weight, developed hoof disease, aborted, and failed to conceive. Milk, beef, pork, eggs, and poultry became contaminated, humans were exposed, and PBB residues were still present in 71 percent of those examined some five years later.

Human Studies. Changes in liver function, an increase in infections, and a decrease in immune functions were observed in study participants having higher levels of PBB in the serum. The majority of those exposed were found to be healthy and to have no symptoms that could be attributed specifically to PBB. Studies are continuing to exclude possible long-term ill-effects from this accidental contamination of food by an industrial poison.

AFLATOXINS

Aflatoxins are a form of naturally occurring mycotoxin found on food as the result of contamination and growth of the yellowish-green molds *Aspergillus flavus and Aspergillus parasiticus.* All are fluorescent substances when exposed to ultraviolet light. They may contaminate foods whenever conditions of temperature and humidity are conducive to the growth of molds.

All farmers and veterinarians and some physicians are knowledgeable about aflatoxins because of their potential danger to animal and human health. Aflatoxin B_1 is recognized as a most potent liver and carcinogenic toxin. In addition, it has mutagenic and teratogenic properties.

Foods affected. Corn and cottonseed meal are most frequently affected. Other foods sometimes contaminated by aflatoxins include peanuts, rice, cereals, soybeans, and peas. Growth of molds may occur in the field or during harvest, storage, processing, shipment, or feeding.

Corn grown in the southeastern United States is most susceptible, and corn from the midwest is 97 percent free from aflatoxin. The maximum allowable limit for animal feed is 20 ppb. Corn produced in southeastern United States has contained more than 20-100 ppb aflatoxin in 30 percent of samples tested.

Disease in Animals. An acute disease in turkeys in England in 1960, causing a loss of 100,000 birds, was linked to aflatoxin-contaminated groundnut meal from Brazil. The concentration of aflatoxin was 10 mg/kg. The birds died of hemorrhages and liver damage. Ducklings, pigs, and calves also ate the contaminated meal and were affected similarly. Newborn animals are more acutely affected than older animals.

Liver carcinomas and kidney tumors develop in various species of animals fed aflatoxins. Rats and trout are the animals most frequently studied for this carcinogenic effect.

Human Liver Cancer. In Thailand, Kenya, Mozambique, Swaziland, and Uganda, the incidence of primary liver cancer has been correlated with the intake of aflatoxin in the diet. A rise in liver cancer incidence is directly related to higher aflatoxin levels in the food and is greater for men than for women. Hepatitis B virus, a common infection in countries with a high incidence of primary liver cancer, may be an additional causative factor.

Cases of *Reye's syndrome* (encephalopathy with fatty degeneration of the liver) might have been caused by aflatoxins in a report from Czechoslovakia. Aspirin is the toxic agent thought to precipitate this illness in children suffering from certain viral diseases in the United States.

An outbreak of epidemic jaundice in India in 1974 was caused by aflatoxins in badly stored maize, heavily contaminated with the fungus, *Aspergillus flavus.* More than 1000 people were affected and the mortality was about one third.

TREMORGENIC MYCOTOXINS

Certain mycotoxins have unusual neurotoxic properties and are named "*tremorgens*." In low doses, they cause whole-body trembling that is sustained for several days in susceptible animals; higher doses are followed by convulsive seizures which may be fatal.

In the United States, various tremorgen-induced syndromes, including paspalum staggers, rye grass staggers, and Bermuda grass tremors, have been described in sheep and cattle. Rye grass staggers in grazing animals is a problem in New Zealand, Australia, and Great Britain.

Tremorgen mycotoxins may also produce disease in humans. A report at the 1992 annual meeting of the Child Neurology Society concerned a Canadian 16 year old boy who had inhaled and/or ingested moulds containing aspergillus fumigatus, flavus and clavitus while helping his father to clean out a silo. The boy was standing at the bottom of the chute and was exposed to the largest dose of mould. He developed fatigue and headache followed by fever, chills and vomiting. His mentation became progressively dulled, and his coordination was incapacitated by a tremor and rigidity of his extremities. He was disorientated, his fund of knowledge was reduced and he could not add two digit numbers. The trembling and symptoms of toxic encephalopathy resolved after seven days and his recovery appeared to be complete. The father who was stationed at the top of the chute, and was exposed to smaller quantities of mould, suffered only mild and transient symptoms of fatigue and headache.

NEPHROTOXIC FUNGI

Ochratoxin A and Citrinin have been isolated from cultures of *Aspergillus and Penicillium* fungi. Naturally occurring levels in edible plants are toxic to the kidneys, and higher levels will damage the liver and intestine of experimental animals. Nephropathy in pigs has been attributed to cereal feed contaminated with ochratoxin.

Citrinin, first studied as an antibiotic, is now a threat to the health of animals and humans as a contaminant of cereals and a kidney toxin.

These nephrotoxic fungi have been implicated as the cause of a chronic progressive kidney disease known as Balkan nephropathy, which occurs endemically in rural populations living along the Danube river.

ESTROGENIC-ANABOLIC FUNGI

Fusarium species form a hormone, Zearalenone, which is found as a natural contaminant of corn and cereals. Pigs fed this hormone-containing food develop an unusual syndrome, *estrogenism.* The syndrome is characterized by enlargement of the vulva and mammary glands and prolapse of the vagina and rectum. The animals become sterile.

Surveys of corn samples in the United States have reported a 15 percent incidence of zearalenone contamination.

Zearalanols are synthesized and used commerc-ially for their anabolic properties, to improve the growth and feed efficiency in sheep and cattle. They have also been tested clinically to relieve menopausal symptoms in women. Their significance as a food toxin in humans is not determined. Future research may show that certain diseases of unknown cause may prove to be related to the mycotoxins in our food.

SWEET POTATO TOXINS

The sweet potato produces stress metabolites, the most abundant being ipomeamarone, that are toxic to animals consuming fungus-infected roots. Reports from the United States and Japan have cited moldy sweet potatoes as the cause of a fatal lung disease of cattle.

In New Guinea the sweet potato is a main dietary item and may account for endemic respiratory diseases among the natives, although the relationship has not yet been proven. Evidence for a health threat to humans from fungus-infected sweet potato is so far lacking.

NITRATES AND NITRITES

Sources in Diet. In addition to the nitrites used as food additives in curing bacon and other pork products (see Chapter 5), humans are exposed to nitrates and nitrites through the drinking water and certain vegetables. The United States Public Health Service allows up to 10 mg/L of nitrate in municipal drinking waters, and this limit is rarely exceeded. Well water may be a source of nitrate poisoning, however.

Cured meats contain about 10 percent of the average daily intake of nitrate in the diet, while the consumption of beets, lettuce, celery, spinach, broccoli, cauliflower, or white potatoes contribute the largest portion of nitrate to the daily diet. Fruits, milk, bread, and water are relatively small sources of the nitrate intake in the diet.

Nitrites formed from nitrates in the saliva account for 75 percent of the daily intake, cured meats contain estimates of 3.5 - 20 percent of the daily nitrite intake, and only 2 percent comes from vegetables.

Purpose of Meat Curing. The addition of nitrite to meats serves three purposes:

1)Antibacterial effect, particularly the inhibition of botulism spores and toxin formation.

2) Formation of pigments responsible for the red or pink color of cured meats; without nitrites, meat would have an unacceptable gray color.

3) Food additive responsible for the safety and stability of cured meats. The level of nitrite permitted in cured meat products in the United States is 200 ppm.

Nitrate-Induced Diseases. Diseases associated with the consumption of nitrates result from the conversion of nitrates to nitrites in the intestine.

Methemoglobinemia. A variety of drugs and chemicals, including acetophenetidin (Phenacetin), aniline based crayons, and nitrites, may increase the rate of oxidation of hemoglobin and produce an acute methemoglobinemia. Newborns are particularly susceptible. The methemoglobin imparts a chocolate brown appearance to the blood and a slate gray cyanotic hue to the skin.

Symptoms of hypoxia may follow, unless the source of nitrite or other chemical is removed. Treatment with an intravenous infusion of methylene blue promotes the rapid conversion of methemoglobin to hemoglobin. An inherited chronic form of methemoglobinemia needs to be considered in the differential diagnosis.

Hot Dog Headache. Nitrite-induced headaches have been reported occasionally in susceptible patients after eating hot dogs, bacon, ham, or salami. The headache is accompanied by flushing of the face and neck, a vasodilator effect of the nitrites.

Stomach Cancer. Humans may be susceptible to the carcinogenic toxicity of nitrates and nitroso compounds formed in the stomach. Significantly higher levels of nitrate have been found in the well waters of regions in Columbia and in two English towns where the incidence of gastric cancer is particularly high. It is speculated that the use of sodium nitrate fertilizer is causally related.

Epidemiological studies suggest that nitrate and/or nitrite may be consumed in meat, vegetables, or drinking water. The nitrate is reduced to nitrite by bacteria in the intestine. Nitrites act on amines in the diet to form nitrosamines, which are carcinogenic. The cancer-inducing health risk of nitrates in the diet is a potential hazard but requires further investigation.

LEAD

Of the major pathways of exposure to lead, food consumption is a large contributor, especially in children. In foods fed to infants, lead is detected in canned evaporated milk and in processed baby formula prepared with some tap waters. The diet of young adults shows higher levels of lead in vegetables and fruits, the daily amount ingested ranging from 90 to 250 mcg.

Metabolism of Lead. The absorption of lead from the intestine depends on the age, nutrition, and health status of the individual. Children absorb 40 percent of ingested lead whereas adults absorb only 10 percent. The physical form of the food is a factor in lead absorption, beverages yielding five to eight times more than solid food.

The lead is first distributed in the blood stream to the various organs of the body, where it accumulates according to the specific affinity of the tissue for lead. The total body lead burden is divided into two main compartments, the soft tissues and bone. The accumulation in bone increases until middle age, whereas lead in soft tissue organs such as liver and kidney remains low and constant and tends to stabilize early in adult life. The lead is excreted in feces, urine, and sweat.

When a person exposed to lead is removed from the source, the half-life of lead in the blood and soft tissues is estimated at 16 days, whereas the half-life of lead in bone is about 16 years. Infants and children, and pregnant females are at greater risk of adverse health effects from lead exposure than other members of the population. Although the World Health Organization has established a provisional tolerable weekly intake for adults of 3 mg lead, no such tolerance level has been documented for infants and children.

For a comprehensive account of lead poisoning, sources of lead, symptoms, and avoidance, see Chapter 1.

MERCURY

Interest in the adverse health effects of mercury has been stimulated by the tragic consequences of environmental contamination of fish and shellfish and the ingestion of bread prepared from wheat accidentally treated with a methylmercurial fungicide.

Mercury in any form entering rivers or bays is converted to methylmercury, the most toxic form, which is then concentrated by fish or other aquatic species in the food chain.

When contaminated fish or shellfish are ingested by humans, the methylmercury passes the blood-brain barrier and produces neurological damage. The high rate of absorption of methylmercury plus the slow rate of excretion potentiates the adverse toxicity.

The exposure of pregnant women is of special concern, since the fetus is especially vulnerable to mercury poisoning. Lactation is an additional hazard because mercury is passed to the infant via breast milk.

Epidemics of methylmercury poisoning have occurred in Japan and Iraq, resulting from industrial waste contamination of water and fungicide treatment of wheat. In the United States, the FDA has conducted a series of surveys of mercury content of food supplies, finding only traces of mercury in shrimp and in the diets of infants and toddlers.

The acidification of rain water, followed by the acidification of lakes and rivers, might cause a change in the concentrations and distribution of a number of toxic metals, including mercury. Acid rain shifts the equilibrium of methylated mercury compounds, favoring the formation of congeners that are concentrated by fish. The potential health problem posed by the mercury in our fish supply requires constant surveillance and avoidance of industrial contamination of our rivers and lakes.

AVOIDANCE OF ENVIRONMENTAL TOXINS

• PCB contamination of the diet can be minimized by avoiding the regular consumption of certain fish, particularly trout and salmon, caught in Lake Michigan, and fish from certain areas of the Hudson river.

•Aflatoxins may be avoided by discarding corn, peanuts, and figs affected by visible mold growth or foods having a moldy taste or odor.

•Nitrates and nitrites may be limited in the diet by washing vegetables and fruit before consumption, reducing the intake of cured meats such as hot dogs and salami, and checking well water for nitrate content.

•Lead ingestion may be reduced to non-hazardous levels by knowledge of the common sources of lead in the environment, and protection of infants and young children from a contaminated water supply or house paint and dust.

•Mercury food poisoning is largely due to accidental contamination and industrial negligence. Recognition of the sources and potential hazards of mercury should serve to heighten public awareness and prevent further contamination of our environment with this toxic element.

Archer MC. Hazards of nitrate, nitrite, and N-nitroso compounds in human nutrition. In: Hathcock JN (ed). Nutritional Toxicology, Vol 1. New York, Academic Press, 1982.

Cordle F, Kolbye AC. Environmental contaminants in food. In: Hathcock JN (ed). Nutritional Toxicology, Vol 1. New York, Academic Press, 1982.

Gordon K, Masotti R, Waddell W. Tremorogenic toxic encephalopathy: a role of mycotoxins in the production of central nervous system disease in humans. Ann Neurol 32; 453: 1992 (abstract).

Henderson WR, Raskin N. Hot dog headache: Individual susceptibility to nitrite. Lancet 2: 1162, 1972.

Jacobson JL, Jacobson SW, Humphrey HEB. Effects of in utero exposure to polychlorinated biphenyls and related contaminants on cognitive functioning in young children. J Pediatr 116:38, 1990.

Lake Michigan Lakewide Management Plan. Chicago, U.S. Environmental Protection Agency, Region V, 1992.

Larone DH. Medically Important Fungi. A Guide to Identification. 2nd Ed. New York, Elsevier Science Publishing Co, 1987.

Wilson BJ. Mycotoxins and toxic stress metabolites of fungus-infected sweet potatoes. In: Hathcock JN (ed). Nutritional Toxicology, Vol 1. New York, Academic Press, 1982.

CHAPTER 8

FOODBORNE INFECTIONS

"Most diseases that man is afflicted with are due to bad foods."

Maimonides, 1135-1204.

Foodborne infections and intoxications are caused by a wide variety of microorganisms, toxins, and chemicals. The incidence of foodborne disease in the United States has been estimated at nine million cases annually. The diagnosis is considered when two or more persons experience a similar illness with gastrointestinal symptoms within 72 hours of ingesting food or water from a common source.

Microorganisms are found in all foods except for soft drinks and foods sterilized by canning. The majority of these microorganisms are harmless to the consumer, but a few species of bacteria may cause infections or intoxications when ingested with food.

Infections occur when small numbers of bacteria enter the body in food and then multiply within the intestine. Intoxications are produced by bacteria that have multiplied and have liberated *exotoxins* into the food before ingestion or *endotoxins* formed within the cell wall of the bacteria after ingestion in food.

The infecting or toxigenic bacteria have well recognized sources and are associated with certain types of foods. The illnesses produced by the bacteria and toxins have different incubation periods and some variation in symptoms which help in the diagnosis. Fortunately, the majority of these infections can be treated and controlled. Hygienic improvements in the production and handling of foods have reduced the frequency of serious outbreaks.

INCUBATION PERIOD AND DIAGNOSIS. The incubation period is a good indication of the cause of the diarrhea. When the time from ingestion of the contaminated food or water to the onset of symptoms is less than one hour, chemical poisoning is the most likely diagnosis. Those outbreaks of diarrhea with incubation periods of one to seven hours are due to enterotoxins formed from *Staphylococcus aureus* or *Bacillus cereus* ; and those of eight to 14 hours incubation are caused by toxins from *Clostridium perfringens.* When symptoms are delayed for more than 14 hours, bacterial infections such as *Salmonella and Shigella, or Norwalk virus* are most commonly involved.

SYMPTOMS AND DIAGNOSIS. Fever and vomiting are the symptoms that help to differentiate the causes of the diarrheal episode. Fever is a rare occurrence in chemical poisoning and toxin-related outbreaks but a common initial symptom in infections due to *Salmonella* and *Shigella.* Vomiting is frequently associated with chemical poisoning and intoxications and only occasionally with infections. Bloody diarrhea without fever is symptomatic of toxic *E. coli* infection.

TABLE 8-1. Clinical Characteristics of Food-borne or Water-borne outbreaks of diarrhea.

Incubation	*Fever*	*Vomiting*	*Cause*
< 1 - 3 hours	Rare	Common	Chemical
1 - 14 hours	Rare	Profuse	Enterotoxins
> 14 hours	Common	Occasional	Infections

INCIDENCE. A total of 954 confirmed outbreaks of foodborne illness was reported to the Centers for Disease Control (CDC), Atlanta, Georgia, in a five year period from various regions of the United States. The cause was bacterial infection or intoxication in 68 percent of cases, and chemical in 24 percent. The actual incidence of foodborne illnesses caused by bacteria is probably unknown, and outbreaks reported to public health authorities may represent only the tip of the iceberg.

The most frequent causes of foodborne outbreaks of diarrheal illness reported to the CDC between 1972 and 1986 are shown in Table 8-2.

TABLE 8-2. Most Frequent Causes of Foodborne Illness Reported to the CDC, 1972-1986, among a Total of 2745 Outbreaks.

Cause	*Percent of Total*
Bacterial	
Salmonella	27
S. aureus	14
C. botulinum	8
C. perfringens	7
Shigella	4
B. cereus	2
V. cholerae	0.2
E. coli	0.1
Chemical	
Ciguatera fish toxin	8
Scromboid fish toxin	7
Mushrooms	2
Heavy metals	2
Shellfish Poisoning (PSP)	1
Chinese Restaurant Syndrome	1
Parasitic	5
Viral	4

Adapted from Mandell GL et al. (eds). Infectious Diseases. 1992.

Salmonella, S. aureus, C. perfringens, and *C. botulinum* were the most frequent bacteria isolated.

Ciguatoxin from fish and mushroom poisoning were the most common chemical causes.

Waterborne outbreaks of diarrhea average 33 per year in the United States and involve approximately 10, 000 people per year.

SOURCES OF INFECTIONS

Foodborne pathogenic bacteria are present in the soil and in animal and human hosts. The reduction or elimination of pathogens from the soil is not possible, but the eradication of sources of infection in animals and in human wastes has provided a safer environment and a reduction in outbreaks of gastrointestinal infection.

Foodborne infections originate from improper storage and handling of food in restaurants in almost half of the epidemic outbreaks of diarrheal illness.

FOOD MISHANDLING. Food prepared commercially for distribution to retailers is subject to strict controls and rigid supervision that ensure a safe supply of food to the consumer. Products are monitored by removal of packages from the processing line for laboratory analysis.

In contrast to the excellent industrial food hygienic practices, foods prepared for consumption at other sites are not under microbiological control. Training in sanitation for kitchen employees may be less than adequate to avoid contamination of food prepared for public consumption.

Outbreaks of foodborne disease occur as the result of mishandling of food in the home and in food service establishments. In addition to restaurants, the kitchens and waiters in hotels, schools, fast food outlets, buffet meal services, churches, weddings, family picnics, camps, colleges, caterers of parties, colleges, nursing homes, hospitals, and other institutions have been indicted as sources of foodborne infections and intoxications.

The most frequently identified food mishandling practices are as follows:

- Improper cooling and inadequate refrigeration of cooked foods.
- Delays in serving from time of preparation.
- Inadequate cooking to destroy pathogens.
- Inadequate reheating of cooked foods.
- Contamination by food handlers and carriers.
- Transfer of pathogens from raw to cooked foods via working counter surfaces, utensils, hands, and aprons.

The use of inadequate heat in cooking and the improper control of refrigeration are the two most frequent factors in the mishandling of food. Foods will unavoidably contain pathogens which are not destroyed in the cooking process and they will be exposed to contamination after cooking. Unless stored in a cold environment, bacteria in food will multiply, resulting in infection or intoxication when consumed.

Principles of Heating Foods. Fluid foods such as soups, stews, and infant formula are heated by convection currents, and the transfer of heat to or from the center, top, or bottom of the container may be hastened by stirring or shaking.

Microwave heating of infant formula is a common practice in the United States, despite concerns of infant scalding. A study of temperature profiles of infant formula in glass and plastic bottles showed that topmost temperatures were significantly higher than temperatures reached at other sites. Routine mixing while microwave heating for 40 - 60 seconds resulted in formula temperatures which could safely be fed to infants. Analysis of riboflavin and vitamin C before and after heating showed no significant loss of nutrient value.

Nonfluid foods such as meat, poultry, and stuffing conduct heat by conduction, according to a principle called *geometry of the mass.* The rate of heat exchange is determined by the thermal conductivity of the food and the surface area of the mass or bird. The interior of large masses may not attain temperatures high enough to kill salmonellae, staphylococci, or other pathogenic organisms. Poultry stuffing heated within the bird are suspect and are more safely cooked separately in shallow pans.

During cooling after cooking, the rate of fall in temperature inside the center of the mass may not be rapid enough to prevent growth of bacteria. Potato and macaroni salads, low acid foods that offer an ideal environment for bacteria, are examples of dishes which require optimal cooking and cooling techniques. All ingredients should be cooked and chilled to prevent growth of bacteria before mixing the final product.

Bacterial Virulence. The virulence of bacteria, their ability to produce disease, varies, and strains within species of bacteria are not uniformally virulent. The ability to produce disease is determined by a "Vi" antigen that is present in certain serotypes of organisms. The presence of bacteriophage and plasmids within the bacterial cell govern the production of enterotoxin and the property of tissue invasiveness and drug resistance. Bacteriophage is a virus that infects bacteria, and plasmids are called "resistance-transfer factors" which change antibiotics to inactive compounds.

Host Susceptibility. Outbreaks of foodborne illness are dependent on the virulence and dose of the pathogenic organism and the susceptibility of the person who ingests the contaminated food.

Both red meats and poultry are contaminated with small numbers of clostridial spores. Under suitable conditions, the spores may germinate and multiply in quantities sufficient to produce disease. Other foods may contain small numbers of pathogenic organisms, even after heating in cooking. The minimum dose of organisms to produce symptoms varies with the susceptibility of the population infected. The infant and geriatric populations are much more susceptible to foodborne infection than the average adult.

FOOD SOURCES OF INFECTIONS AND TOXINS

Salmonella outbreaks follow the ingestion of poultry, beef, eggs, or dairy products. The role of raw, unpasteurized or contaminated milk has been emphasized in several recent epidemics. Eggs and chocolate have also been the sources of large outbreaks of *Salmonella* infection.

Shigella outbreaks occur with servings of potato and egg salads. The cool and moist state of these foods are conducive to bacterial contamination and proliferation. Raw vegetables served at a salad bar were the vehicle for *Shigella* dysentery in a recent outbreak.

Staphylococcal food poisoning is associated with ham, poultry, egg and potato salads, and cream-filled pastries. These foods are contaminated by food handlers who harbor the organism in the nose and on the hands. The symptoms are due to preformed enterotoxins.

Bacillus cereus food poisoning of the short-incubation type has been traced to fried rice that has been cooked and kept warm for extended periods. The powdered milk in macaroni and cheese was the source of infection in one reported outbreak due to *B. cereus.*

Long-incubation *B. cereus* outbreaks occur when certain foods are prepared in large quantities for banquets or in institutions, and when the food is stored and is not reheated satisfactorily at the time of serving. "Meals-on-wheels," providing food held at or above room temperature for long periods, is another source of *B. cereus* epidemics. The foods contaminated include meats, vegetables, milk products, and dried beans, cereals, seasonings, spices, and potatoes.

Clostridium perfringens has been isolated in outbreaks following the ingestion of beef, poultry, gravies, and fish, improperly stored and inadequately heated at the time of serving.

Clostridium botulinum, an anaerobic spore-forming bacillus that produces neurotoxins and the symptoms of botulism, may contaminate low-acid foods (that is, those with a pH > 4.6), such as home-canned vegetables, fruits, and fish. Recent outbreaks of botulism have followed the ingestion of baked potatoes, sauteed onions, and chopped garlic. Honey is the most common source of botulism in infants.

Commercially canned foods are subject to high standards and have an excellent record of safety. Canned meats and salami and sausages are preserved by adding salt and nitrate to inhibit the growth of *C. botulinum* spores. Acidic fruits (pH < 4.6) and acidified vegetables are subjected to pasteurization and depend on the low pH to inhibit the production of botulinum toxin.

Some fruits such as tomatoes may harbor aerobic spore-bearing bacteria and yeasts that alter the pH and permit the growth of *C. botulinum* spores. If canned food is contaminated, the container will be blown.

The use of *modified atmosphere packaging* and the dependence on refrigeration to extend the shelf life of raw meat, fresh fish, and processed foods without preservatives carry a potential risk of botulism from these products. Coleslaw prepared from shredded cabbage kept in a modified atmosphere packaging which excludes air and oxygen has been linked to four cases of botulism. Toxin was detected within four days after inoculation of the shredded cabbage with *C. botulinum* spores.

Mushrooms stored in sealed containers contaminated with *C. botulinum* spores develop botulinum toxin. Toxin formation is prevented if oxygen is introduced in the package. The Food and Drug Administration recommends packaging of mushrooms in containers pierced with air holes to prevent the formation of botulinum toxin.

Vacuum packaging may be conducive to the growth of anaerobic organisms such as *C. botulinum,* and toxin may be produced at room temperatures or possibly at refrigeration temperature. Additional safety controls, including heat treatment after packaging, inoculation with lactic acid bacilli, and low dose irradiation have been considered.

In Europe, where modified atmosphere packaging has been used for several years, no case of botulism has been attributed to this form of food storage.

Vibrio cholerae outbreaks have been traced to the ingestion of contaminated shellfish, including crabs, shrimp, and raw oysters. These infections are rare and have been reported particularly in Guam and in Louisiana in the United States.

Travelers' diarrhea caused by *Escherichia coli* infection is associated with the consumption of salads, undercooked meat and other foods, water, and ice in developing countries where diarrhea is hyperendemic. Enterotoxigenic *E. coli* is the most commonly identified cause of travelers' diarrhea, but a variety of bacteria, viruses, and parasites may be involved.

Bloody diarrhea and kidney failure, a *hemorrhagic colitis-uremic syndrome* that may be fatal, occurs with some toxic *E. coli* foodborne infections.

SOURCES OF CHEMICAL POISONING

Ciguatera fish poisoning has been associated with over 400 species of fish. Grouper is the most frequently identified source of the ciguatoxin, and barracuda, red snapper, amberjack, and dolphin have also been implicated.

Ciguatoxin and maitotoxin occur in high concentrations in a dinoflagellate microscopic organism found along coral reefs. This organism is ingested by small fish and the toxin is absorbed and concentrated in the fish flesh and muscles. Larger fish consume the smaller fish, and the toxin is absorbed from the gastrointestinal tract and is again concentrated in the musculature. The passsage of the toxin along the food chain results in the accumulation of large and poisonous concentrations in the fish eaten by humans.

Scombroid (pseudoallergic) fish poisoning has occurred after ingestion of tuna, mackerel, and kingfish. The nonscombroid fish, mahi-mahi, has also caused outbreaks of scombroid-like fish poisoning.

Paralytic Shellfish Poisoning is caused by eating mussels, clams, oysters, and sea scallops contaminated during dinoflagellate blooms, or "red tides."

Outbreaks of *heavy metal poisoning*, caused by cadmium, copper, iron, and tin, have been associated with acidic beverages, including lemonade, fruit punch, and carbonated drinks, that have been stored in corroded metalic containers or punch bowls. Vending machines and metallic tubing may also be implicated.

EPIDEMIOLOGY

Factors which determine the frequencies and distributions of foodborne infections and intoxications include seasonality and geographic location. The time of year of an epidemic may provide a pointer to the cause of the outbreak. Bacterial infections such as *S. aureus, Salmonella,* and *Shigella* are common during the summer months. *C. perfringens* outbreaks occur throughout the year but are least frequent during the summer. *Botulism* is more common during the summer and fall.

Chemical food poisoning shows some seasonal variability in incidence. Paralytic shellfish poisoning, which is related to a red tide, is most common in the summer and fall. Ciquatera outbreaks occur in the spring and summer. Mushroom poisoning is most common in the spring, late summer, and the fall.

Geographic location of the outbreak is important in diagnosis. *V. cholerae* infection in the United States occurs chiefly on the Gulf Coast. Some outbreaks of *botulism* are common to the west of the Mississippi River, some occur in the East of the United States, and others are common to the Great Lakes Region, depending on the organism type, A, B, or E.

Over 90 percent of outbreaks of ciquatera in the United States have been reported from Florida and Hawaii. Ciquatera is also common in the West Indies. Paralytic shellfish poisoning occurs in coastal areas of Florida, New England, and California.

The identification of the food vehicle in a food-borne outbreak of diarrhea requires analysis of food-specific attack rates for all foods and beverages served at the banquet or meal. A food must have a significantly higher attack rate for those persons who ate it than for those who did not. To be incriminated in the outbreak, the food should have been eaten by most of those persons who became ill.

LABORATORY DIAGNOSIS

The appropriate laboratory specimens required for the confirmation of the cause of a food-borne outbreak are obtained from the patient, the food handler, the food specimens, and the food-preparation environment.

The patient specimens include stools, vomitus, and blood for culture and serotyping of organisms, and assay of enterotoxins. Food handlers are examined for evidence of the offending organism on the hands, in nasal secretions, and in the stools.

Outbreaks of food poisoning may be confirmed by the isolation of the organism of the same type from vomitus or feces of ill people, the food, and from the skin of the food handler. The demonstration of enterotoxin in the food and the serum or stool of ill people is also employed in the laboratory analysis.

Food is analysed for metallic ions when heavy metal poisoning is suspected. Ciquatera outbreaks are diagnosed by the clinical manifestations of the illness, and the demonstration of ciquatoxin in the incriminated fish. Scombroid fish poisoning may be confirmed by an estimation of histamine concentration in the fish; 100 mg per 100 g of fish flesh correlates with toxicity. Shellfish poisoning may be confirmed by finding the toxin in mollusks or elevated quantities of dinoflagellate in the sea water.

Mushroom poisoning is diagnosed by the symptoms, and the demonstration of toxin in gastric contents, blood, urine, or stools. Chinese restaurant syndrome may be confirmed by analysis of the food for elevated concentrations of monosodium glutamate.

More than 50 per cent of the reported foodborne disease outbreaks in the United States are of undetermined cause.

SPECIFIC INFECTIONS AND TOXINS

SALMONELLOSES

The salmonellae are the most ubiquitous group of microorganisms that cause foodborne or waterborne diarrhea. In humans, salmonella infection occurs in three forms: 1) Enteric fever, such as typhoid or paratyphoid fever, 2) Acute gastroenteritis, the most common form, and 3) Focal infections causing osteomyelitis and abscess formation.

Salmonella typhi , causing typhoid fever, and *S. paratyphi* A and B, the agents of paratyphoid fever, affect only humans and are not natural pathogens for animals. Typhoid fever is now rare in the United States but is a serious disease, with a fatality rate of 12 - 25 per cent before the advent of antibiotics. A carrier state is common after recovery from the acute bacteremia and fever, and the organism establishes permanent residence in the gallbladder without harm to the host. Surgical removal of the gallbladder is often required to make the patient carrier-free.

Typhoid bacteria are transmitted to foods by the hands of carriers, insects, rodents, and water contaminated with infected human wastes. Shellfish grown in polluted water and nonrefrigerated milk are frequent sources of infection. Improved hygiene, education regarding methods of avoiding foodborne infection, immunization of persons travelling to endemic areas, and proper treatment of human sewage have reduced the incidence of enteric fevers in the United States.

SALMONELLA FOOD POISONING

Salmonella typhimurium and S. enteritidis are the two earliest species of salmonella bacteria to be described. More than 1800 different serotypes of *S. enteritidis* have been isolated, but 10 salmonella serotypes account for 75 percent of clinical outbreaks of salmonella food poisoning. Identification of serotypes is important in epidemiology and in recognition of the common source of infection in outbreaks.

These salmonella organisms are pathogenic to animals and humans. Their widespread dissemination in the food-processing industry, and particularly in egg and poultry production, explains the high frequency of infection among the populations of the United States and other countries.

Poultry growers use feeds containing animal by-products that are infected with salmonellae. The salmonellae multiply in the gastrointestinal tracts of the birds, contaminate the surface of their eggs, and persist in the poultry flesh after evisceration. The Department of Agriculture in the United States has recently issued a warning that eggs should be kept refrigerated to minimize the danger of salmonellosis in the consumer. Packages of eggs will need to carry a label to this effect by the year 1994.

If eggs are stored at room temperature, salmonellae pass through the shell and contaminate the egg albumin within three days. Cracked eggs are a major hazard and should be used only in dishes requiring cooking at temperatures sufficient to destroy the organisms. Soft-boiled eggs and Eggs-Benedict have been removed from the menu in some restaurants and hotels.

The list of foods incriminated as vehicles in outbreaks of salmonella food poisoning includes the following: Poultry, eggs, ham, turkey, meat loaf, pork sausage, and fish or shellfish.

Between the years 1955 and 1985, the number of cases of salmonellosis reported annually in the United States has increased steadily from 4 per 100,000 population to 27 per 100,000. The highest incidence was in children less than 10 years of age. The relatively low infection rate after 10 years suggests the development of immunity to salmonella in adults, except for those over 70 years of age.

Prevention. Salmonellosis may be avoided by following certain well-established principles of food selection and preparation.

- Avoid all raw meats and animal-derived raw foods in the diet.
- Educate food handlers in optimal methods of personal and workplace sanitation.
- Prevent cross-contamination of prepared or cooked foods with raw foods by cleaning and disinfecting all working surfaces and utensils used in handling raw foods.

- Avoid use of aprons as towels and handkerchiefs while preparing raw food.
- Maintain separate working areas for raw foods.
- Eggs should be washed and stored refrigerated.

STAPHYLOCOCCUS ENTEROINTOXICATION

Staphylococcus aureus is the second most frequent cause of outbreaks of foodborne disease in the United States. Outbreaks are often associated with large gatherings at which readily formulated foods are served.

The staphylococcal organism lives in the nose and pharynx. It is distributed widely in droplets during coughing, sneezing, and by touching the lips while smoking and by blowing the nose. "Catching a sneeze" with the palm of the hand collects 5000 staphylococci/cm^2 on the skin. Skin infections are another source of *S. aureus* in food handlers that have been found responsible for some outbreaks of enterointoxication.

S. aureus produces six enterotoxins, A through F. Type A has been responsible for more than 50 percent of staphylococcal food poisoning in the United States. The toxins are only partially inactivated by even prolonged boiling, and they are resistant to the amount of heat usually employed in cooking foods. The toxins in food may be isolated by immunological tests, including hemagglutinin inhibition, and radioimmunoassay.

Symptoms. Only small amounts of toxin are needed to produce symptoms. The severity of the diarrhea, vomiting, and abdominal cramps is correlated with the amount of toxin consumed. Fever is not a characteristic feature of staphylococcal intoxication.

Food Sources. Any food prepared and handled after cooking can be contaminated with staphylococcal toxin. Foods incriminated have been heated and cooled, and provide a favorable environment for bacterial growth and toxin formation. Legal limits of contamination restrict the number of staphylococci to 100 per gram of food.

Ham, poultry, custards, meringues, pumpkin pies, and cream pies may be contaminated on the surface during cooling, if a temperature above 10°C is maintained for more than four hours. Meat, poultry, seafood salads, macaroni salad, icings, cake fillers, whipped cream, filled cakes and pastries, and sandwiches, foods which are prepared with cooked or heated ingredients, are further categories known to harbor the toxin. Safe preparation of such foods demands the cooling of all ingredients to or below 10°C before formulation.

Prevention. The following three simple measures should be observed to reduce or prevent foodborne staphylococcal intoxication:

- Avoid types of foods susceptible to staphylococcal contamination when eating at gatherings where poor hygiene is suspected.
- Educate food handlers in approved personal hygiene habits to lower the risk of contamination.
- Maintain foods at <10°C during storage and for not more than four hours in the temperature range of 10 - 50°C while serving.

BOTULISM

Of 721 outbeaks of botulism in the United States during a 76-year period, 65 were connected to commercially processed foods and 519 to home-canned foods. The origins of the remaining cases were unknown. In recent years, commercial sources have been rare, but home-processed foods have continued to be incriminated. The serving of home-canned foods in public restaurants and stores is now prohibited.

Clostridium botulinum produces seven types of toxin. Types A and B, the most common, are found in red meats and vegetables, and E and F toxins are the cause of botulism that follows the consumption of uncooked, salted, smoked, or pickled fish and fish eggs. Type G is a rare cause in humans, and types C and D affect only poultry, cattle and horses.

Botulinum toxins are inactivated by heating at 80°C for 30 minutes. Spores of *C. botulinum* are destroyed by heat at 121°C for two and one-half minutes, but many foods cannot withstand this temperature. Canned foods such as cured meats, including hams, luncheon meats, frankfurters, and sausages, are subjected to heat below that necessary to sterilize the food, and growth of spores is inhibited by the addition of nitrite and salt. Acidic fruits and vegetables are treated by pasteurization, and the low pH inhibits toxin production.

Botulism in children and adults is caused by the ingestion of preformed toxin. Infantile botulism, often related to honey used to sweeten the formula, results from ingestion of spores in the honey and subsequent production of the toxin in the intestine. Both forms of intoxication last for several weeks to months. Clinical suspicion is critical in arriving at an early diagnosis.

Symptoms of Botulism. Symptoms of botulinum intoxication may present within six hours of ingestion of the toxin. Usually, symptoms are delayed for 12-36 hours. Typically, the muscles supplied by the cranial nerves are affected first. Ninety percent of patients suffer from blurred vision, 76 percent have swallowing difficulties, and 50 percent complain of generalized weakness, nausea and vomiting, and slurred speech. Less frequent symptoms and signs include drooping eyelids, pupil changes, abdominal pain, diarrhea or constipation, bladder disturbances, and drowsiness. Consciousness is not impaired.

Diagnosis. Acute gastrointestinal symptoms occurring simultaneously with visual blurring and a descending paralysis suggest the diagnosis of foodborne botulism. Toxin may not be detected in the blood, stomach contents, and stools. The diagnosis is usually made on clinical grounds.

The transmission of nerve impulses is impaired due to the block of acetylcholine release by botulinum neurotoxin. Electromyographic testing will confirm the neuromuscular site of toxin damage, but EMG responses may be atypical, particularly in the early stages of the illness.

Patients suspected of having botulism are observed in hospital, and a public health enquiry is conducted to detect possible sources of food contamination. New techniques for preserving foods have increased the risks of occurrence of botulism and require a greater awareness of the diagnostic signs.

Consumer confidence in the new methods of food production would be improved by the development of reliable, time-temperature indicators for refrigerated processed foods and for fresh foods sold in modified atmosphere packaging. Botulism can be prevented by careful attention to food preparation and storage.

PERFRINGENS GASTROENTERITIS

Clostridium perfringens is found in soil and in the intestinal tract of humans and animals. It is ubiquitous in the home and kitchen and in many foods. Spore formation in the intestinal tract results in the release of the toxin.

Sources of this foodborne intoxication include beef, pork, and poultry, and stews and soups containing these meats. Meats are poor conductors of heat. The larger the piece of meat, or the larger the pot of stew, the more prolonged the cooling period and the time during which the organism can multiply.

Foods kept more than four hours after cooking must be refrigerated rapidly to avoid the risk of dangerous levels of *C. perfringens.* If refrigeration is inadequate, meat must be reheated to a minimum of 63°C before serving. Many of the outbreaks of intoxication have resulted from the roasting of large joints of beef and the serving of leftovers on the following day, without optimal refrigeration or reheating.

Symptoms. The illness is often mild but may affect large numbers of individuals in a single outbreak. Symptoms rarely persist for more than 12-24 hours. Abdominal cramps, diarrhea, and gas are the most prominent symptoms. Fever, dehydration, and headache are rare.

Prevention. Large joints of meat should be cooked only if the kitchen and dining facilities permit immediate serving or adequate cooling and storage of meat leftovers. Recommendations for the institutional handling of beef served in restaurants should be followed explicitly to prevent outbreaks of perfringens gastroenteritis.

BACILLUS CEREUS INTOXICATION

Gastroenteritis produced by *B. cereus* is similar to that of *C. perfringens* intoxication. Symptoms develop within 10 hours of ingestion of contaminated food and persist for 10 hours. Abdominal pain, diarrhea, headache, and dizziness are the main symptoms. Fever and vomiting are less common.

Sources of this foodborne intoxication include starchy foods such as fried and cooked rice, leftover reconstituted potatoes, bean sprouts, and meat dishes. Living bacteria in high numbers are essential for intoxication to occur. Outbreaks are more common in Europe than in the United States.

Prevention. Food preparation should conform to the following principles:

- Prompt refrigeration of foods not served immediately after cooking.
- Foods inadequately cooled must be reheated to 60°C to destroy bacteria before serving.

SHIGELLOSIS

Shigellosis is a disease of the large bowel. It has an incubation period of one to seven days. Symptoms include abdominal pain, fever, frequent watery and sometimes bloody diarrhea, and occasionally vomiting and dehydration. Four different clinical syndromes are recognized:

1) Asymptomatic excretion of shigella organism,
2) Enterotoxin-like diarrhea,
3) Bacillary dysentery, and
4) Arthritic syndrome.

There are four serogroups of *Shigella* with over 40 serotypes. *S. sonnei* is the most common cause of bacillary dysentery in the United States and Europe. *S. flexneri,* the Flexner bacillus, and *S. boydii,* the Boyd bacillus, are uncommon causes. *S. dysenteriae* , a severe form, is endemic in the Far East and is rarely encountered in the United States.

Shigellae are chiefly waterborne. Children under 10 years of age are at greatest risk. Foods were incriminated in only eight of 366 outbreaks reported in one publication in 1972. These included chocolate pudding, tossed salad, turkey salad, spaghetti, and poi. The last item was served at a Hawaiian wedding reception and caused shigellosis in 1000 guests. Tuna salad and food from a salad bar, contaminated by a cafeteria worker, caused an outbreak at a hospital which involved 280 employees and visitors.

Foods become contaminated directly by handlers who are suffering from shigellosis or by those who are carriers of the organism. Exposure to contaminated water is another source of infection. Shigellosis is a disease of humans, and is spread via fecal contamination of food or water. Animals are not affected. It is often a disease of poverty and occurs frequently under wartime conditions, when optimal sanitation is disrupted.

Prevention. 1) Sanitary collection and treatment of human sewage, and 2) careful supervision of food handlers in the practice of personal hygiene.

CIGUATERA FISH POISONING

The onset of symptoms is rapid, usually within 2-30 hours. The earliest symptoms are diarrhea, vomiting, and abdominal pain. A later and second phase of illness includes muscle pain, and a disturbed hot and cold sensation around the mouth and in the limbs.

Treatment. Intravenous fluids may be required for dehydration. Mannitol is sometimes used for treatment of coma and other neurological manifestations of intoxication.

Symptoms may continue for as long as three weeks, and are usually self-limiting.

SCOMBROID FISH POISONING

The onset of symptoms is within 10 minutes to two hours following ingestion. Diarrhea, nausea, and abdominal pain are accompanied by histamine-related symptoms, including flushing of the skin, sweating, urticaria, facial swelling, burning sensation around the mouth, dizziness, and respiratory distress.

Treatment. Gastric lavage decreases absorption of histamine. Intravenous fluids may be required for dehydration. Antihistamines are sometimes beneficial. Cimetidine, a histamine-blocker, has been successful in severe cases.

Symptoms are usually self-limiting. Recovery is expected in 10 hours.

PARALYTIC SHELLFISH POISONING

The onset of symptoms is acute, and occurs within one-half to two hours after ingestion. Numbness and tingling sensations around the mouth and in the hands and feet are the most common complaints. Ataxic gait, vertigo, and paralysis of the diaphragm with respiratory distress occur less frequently. A floating sensation can be characteristic.

Treatment. No known antidote is available. Mechanical ventilation for respiratory paralysis may be required.

Symptoms are usually self-limiting, but weakness may persist for weeks.

MUSHROOM POISONING

Four clinical syndromes and seven types of toxin are associated with wild mushroom poisoning:

- *Gastrointestinal- Delayed Onset.* Amanita poisoning.
- *Autonomic Nervous System.* Muscarine type.
- *Central Nervous System.* Ibotenic acid and Muscimol.
- *Gastrointestinal- Rapid Onset.* Various toxins.

The toxins produced by wild mushrooms are cyclopeptides, monomethylhydrazine, muscarine, coprine, ibotenic acid, psilocybin, and unknown types.

Amanita Poisoning. Poisoning from *Amanita* and *Galerina* species accounts for 95 percent of the fatalities from mushroom intoxication. The mortality rate for amanita poisoning is reported at 5-10 percent.

Symptoms develop in two phases: 1) Within six to 24 hours following ingestion, nausea, vomiting, and abdominal pain are followed by profuse, watery diarrhea; 2) Symptoms delayed for 24-48 hours include jaundice, liver dysfunction, renal failure, and coma. A low prothrombin time is a sign of a poor prognosis, and death may occur within four to seven days.

Treatment is supportive and specific. Dehydration is corrected by fluid replacement, and aspiration of duodenal contents will decrease the toxin load. The effects of amanitotoxin may be blocked by intravenous penicillin and silibinin.

Monomethylhydrazine intoxication, another form of gastrointestinal-delayed onset, mushroom poisoning, is characterized by the inhibition of gamma-aminobutyric acid and methemoglobinemia. Treatment includes intravenous pyridoxine and methylene blue.

Muscarine Poisoning. This autonomic nervous system, rapid onset, form of mushroom poisoning results from toxins that bind to postsynaptic receptors and produce an exaggerated cholinergic response.

Symptoms are of rapid onset, and consist of sweating, tearing, salivation, small pupils, incontinence, bronchospasm, increased pulmonary secretion, and vomiting.

Treatment consists of atropine sulfate, the specific antidote, administered intravenously until the respiratory symptoms resolve.

Muscimol Intoxication. Muscimol, a hallucinogen, and ibotenic acid, an insecticide, are contained in *Amanita muscaria* and *Amanita pantherina* . These toxins have anticholinergic effects. They cause a central nervous system, rapid onset, form of mushroom poisoning.

Hallucinations and euphoria occur within one half to two hours following ingestion. Vomiting, seizures, and coma develop with large doses of the toxins. If muscarine is also present, symptoms of an exaggerated cholinergic response will occur.

Specific therapy is selected according to the type of cholinergic symptoms. Atropine is given if an exaggerated cholinergic response is predominant. Physostigmine is used to reverse the delirium caused by the anticholinergic effects of muscimol.

"Magic mushrooms" contain psilocybin and psilocin, two psychotropic compounds that cause euphoria and hallucinations. Severely agitated patients respond to diazepam. Symptoms resolve within six hours.

Gastrointestinal - Rapid Onset Syndrome. Many mushrooms with toxins of unknown types may cause a rapid onset, gastrointestinal syndrome that must be differentiated from the amanita poisoning of delayed onset and more serious prognosis.

Symptoms develop within an hour of ingestion and last from hours to days. They consist of abdominal pain, nausea, vomiting, and diarrhea. Treatment is largely supportive, and no specific therapy is known.

Aronoff SC. Food poisoning. In: Behrman RE(ed),Nelson Textbook of Pediatrics, 14th Ed, Philadelphia, WB Saunders, 1992.

Hughes JM, Tauxe RV. Food-borne disease. In: Mandell GL, Douglas RG Jr, Bennett JE (eds). Principles and Practice of Infectious Diseases, 3rd Ed, New York, Churchill Livingstone, 1990.

Hutchinson DN. Foodborne botulism. BMJ 305:264, 1992.

Mundt JO. Hazards of foodborne bacterial infections and intoxications. In: Hathcock JN (ed). Nutritional Toxicology Vol I, New York, Academic Press, 1982.

Pickering LK, Cleary TG. Gastrointestinal infections. In: Feigin RD, Cherry JD. Textbook of Pediatric Infectious Diseases, 2nd ed, Vol 1 & 2. Philadelphia, WB Sauders, 1987.

Sigman-Grant M, Bush G, Anantheswaran R. Microwave heating of infant formula: a dilemma resolved. Pediatrics 90: 412, 1992.

Sommers HM, Shulman ST. In: Shulma ST, Phair JP, Sommers HM. (eds). The Biological and Clinical Basis of Infectious Diseases, 4th ed. Philadelphia, WB Saunders, 1992.

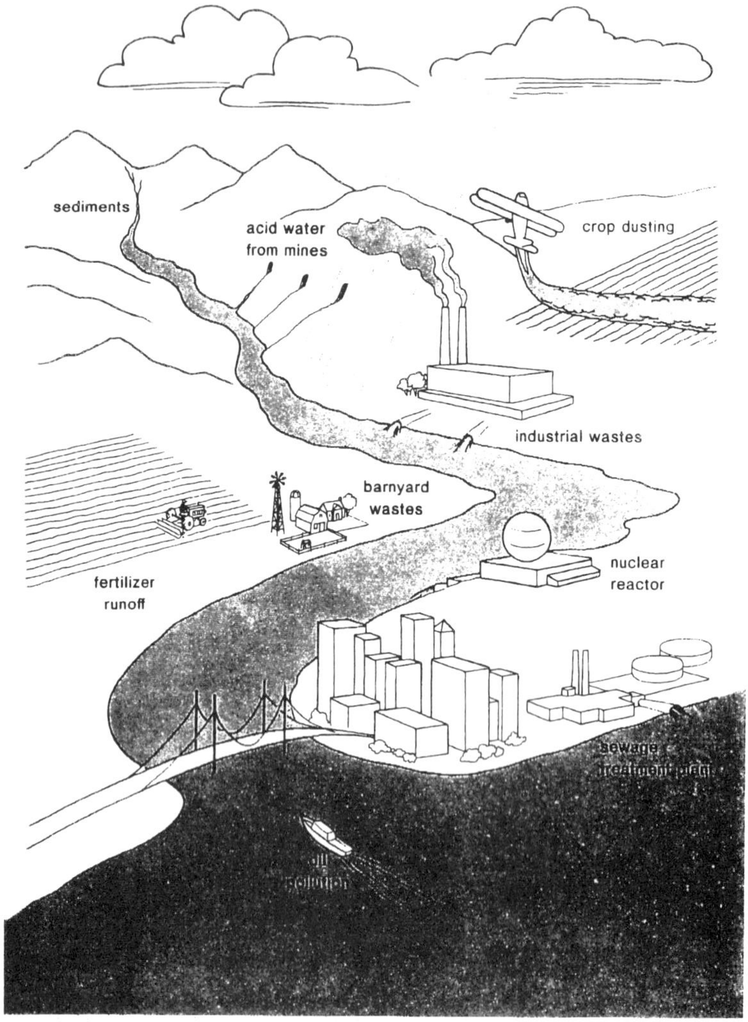

Figure 9-1. Showing sources of water pollution from industrial wastes, fertilizer runoff, crop dusting, nuclear reactor, and sewage treatment plant.

Reproduced and adapted from U.S. Environmental Protection Agency, Office of Water Supply and Solid Waste Management Programs, "Waste Disposal Practices and Their Effects on Ground Water" Executive Summary, (Washington, D.C., U.S. Government Printing Office, 1977).

CHAPTER 9

WATERBORNE DISEASES

"And let this be the law: If anyone intentionally pollutes the water of another...by poisonous substances, whether the water of a spring, or collected in reservoirs, ...let the injured party bring the cause before the warden of the city."

Plato, 427-347 B.C.

Organisms that cause waterborne outbreaks of disease differ in type and frequency from those responsible for foodborne outbreaks. The causative agents for waterborne disease outbreaks reported to the Centers for Disease Control, Atlanta, USA, 1972 through 1985, are shown in Table 9-1.

Giardia lamblia was the pathogenic agent most frequently recognized in the United States. It accounted for 85 outbreaks in the 14 year period and almost 40 percent of the total number reported. The majority of waterborne disease is of unknown cause.

Coliform bacteria from human and animal wastes are found in drinking water if the water is not treated properly. These bacteria may cause disease themselves or may be an indication that other harmful organisms may be present in the water supply. Waterborne diseases such as typhoid, cholera, infectious hepatitis, and dysentery have been traced to improperly disinfected drinking water.

TABLE 9-1. Most Frequent Defined Causes of Waterborne Disease Outbreaks Reported to the CDC, 1972-1985.

Cause	*Percent of Total*
G. lamblia	39
Shigella	12
Hepatitis A	8
Norwalk-like agents	7
C. jejuni	5
Salmonella	5
S. typhi	2
Various organisms	2
Miscellaneous chemicals	20

Adapted from Mandell GL et al. Infectious Diseases, 1990.

DRINKING WATER STANDARDS

Most substances currently regulated under the **Safe Drinking Water Act** (1974) occur naturally in our environment and in the foods we eat. The regulations set levels of drinking water quality to protect our health. They were originally called "interim" regulations because the 1974 Act stipulated that the Environmental Protection Agency (EPA) was to issue Maximum Contaminant Levels (MCLs) on an interim basis and revise them periodically.

The 1986 amendments to the Act require EPA to issue a MCL Goal (MCLG) as well as an MCL. An MCLG is an unenforceable health goal equal to the maximum level of a contaminant not expected to cause adverse health effects over a lifetime of exposure.

As an alternative to the MCLG, the EPA can adopt a "National Primary Drinking Water Regulation" that requires the use of a specific treatment method be used to control a contaminant. The Agency uses this option when it is not technically or economically feasible to determine how much of a contaminant is present in drinking water.

The EPA National Primary Drinking Water Standards for 30 contaminants are shown in Table 9-2. Only two substances for which standards have been set pose an immediate threat to health whenever they are exceeded: 1) Bacteria, and 2) Nitrate.

Bacteria. If the coliform count in our water exceeds the standard level of safety, we should receive notice and directions to be followed to protect our health.

TABLE 9-2. National Primary Drinking Water Standards.

Contaminants	*Health Effects*	*MCL*	*Sources*
Organic Chemicals			
Acrylamide	cancer, nervous	TT	sewage
Alachlor	cancer	.002	herbicide
Aldicarb	nervous system	.003	insecticide
Atrazine	cardiac	.003	herbicide
Benzene	cancer	.005	fuel, solvent
Carbofuran	reproduction	.04	insecticide
Carbon tetraCl	cancer	.005	coolants
Chlordane	cancer	.002	insecticide
2,4-D	liver, kidney, cns	.07	herbicide
DiBrClpropane	cancer	.0002	fumigant
DiClbenzene	cancer	.075	moth balls
DiClbenzene o-	cns, lung, liver	.6	solvent
Dichloroethane	cancer	.005	insecticides
DiClethylene	liver, kidney	.007	dyes, paints
DiClethylene(cis)	cns, liver	.07	solvent
DiClethylene(trans)	cns, liver	.1	solvent
DiClpropane	cancer, liver	.005	fumigant
Endrin	cns, kidney	.0002	insecticide
EpiClhydrin	cancer, liver	TT	epoxy resin
Ethylbenzene	kidney, liver	.7	gasoline
Ethylene DiBromide	cancer	.00005	gasoline
Heptachlor	cancer	.0004	insecticide
Lindane	cns, liver	.0002	insecticide
Methoxychlor	cns, liver	.04	insecticide
MonoClbenzene	kidney, liver	.1	pesticide
PentaClphenol	cancer, liver	.001	herbicide
PCBs	cancer	.0005	transformer

TABLE 9-2 continued (Adapted from U.S. EPA Report, 1991)

Organic Chemicals			
Styrene	liver, cns	.1	plastics
TetraClethylene	cancer	.005	solvent
Toluene	kidney, cns	1	gasoline
Trihalomethanes	cancer	.1	Cl water
Toxaphene	cancer	.003	insecticide
Silvex 2-4-5TP	cns, liver	.05	herbicide
TriClethane	nervous system	.2	food wraps
TriClethylene	cancer	.005	paints
Vinyl chloride	cancer	.002	pipes
Xylenes	liver, kidney	10	paint, ink
Inorganic Chemicals			
Arsenic	skin, nervous	.05	pesticide
Asbestos	cancer	7 MFL	pipes
Barium	blood	2	paint
Cadmium	kidney	.005	plumbing
Chromium	liver, skin, gi	.1	textiles
Copper	gastrointestinal	TT	plumbing
Fluoride	bones	4	additive
Lead	cns, kidney	.05	plumbing
Mercury	kidney, cns	.002	fungicide
Nitrate	"blue-baby"	10	fertilizer
Selenium	nervous system	.05	mining
Radionuclides	cancer		nuclear waste
Microbiological			
Giardia lamblia	Giardiasis		fecal matter
Legionella	Legionnaires		aerosols
Coliforms	gi disease risk		fecal matter
Viruses	gastroenteritis		fecal matter

MCL, mg/L; TT, treatment required; cns, nervous system.

Nitrate. Nitrate in drinking water above the national standard poses an immediate threat to children six months to one year old. Excessive levels of nitrate may react with the hemoglobin in the blood to produce an anemic condition commonly known as "blue baby."

If a notice of excessive quantities of nitrate in the drinking water is received, do not give the water to infants under three months of age and do not use it to prepare the infant formula. The water should not be boiled, since this will increase the nitrate concentr-ation.

In addition to the MCLs, the effects on our health and the sources of each contaminant are listed in the EPA report (1991). Bacteria and nitrate in levels exceeding the MCLs are an immediate danger to our health. The remaining 28 contaminants may prove harmful if the MCLs are exceeded over long periods of time.

Secondary Drinking Water Standards are federal guidelines regarding the aesthetic quality of the water, such as taste, odor, and color. Water with these contaminants above the Secondary Maximum Contaminant Level (SMCL) may not be pleasant to drink, but it will not cause health problems. The EPA provides these standards as guidelines to the States and as reasonable goals. Federal law does not require water systems to comply with them. States may choose to enforce them, however.

The effects of 13 contaminants for which the EPA has developed Secondary Drinking Water Standards as guidelines for the States are shown in Table 9-3.

TABLE 9-3. EPA Secondary Drinking Water Standards.

Contaminants	***Levels***	***Effects***
Aluminum	.05-.2 mg/L	discoloration
Chloride	250 mg/L	taste; corrosion
Color	15 units	aesthetic
Copper	1 mg/L	taste; staining
Corrosivity	non-corrosive	leaching lead
Fluoride	2 mg/L	brown teeth
Foaming agents	.5 mg/L	aesthetic
Iron	.3 mg/L	taste; staining
Manganese	.05 mg/L	taste; staining
Odor	3 threshold	aesthetic
pH	6.5-8.5	corrosion
Silver	.1 mg/L	discolored skin
Sulfate	250 mg/L	taste; laxative
Total solids (TDS)	500 mg/L	taste; corrosion
Zinc	5 mg/L	taste

Adapted from US EPA Publication, September 1991.

The Safe Drinking Water Act of 1974 gave the United States its first comprehensive national program to safeguard public drinking water. It established the national drinking water standards, which protect the health of everyone who receives their drinking water from systems serving at least 25 people or having at least 15 service connections. More than 80 percent of the U.S. population and a quarter million drinking water systems, including non-community water systems, are affected by the Act.

The amendments to the Act, introduced in 1986, issued deadlines to the EPA for specifying criteria for the filtration of surface water supplies and the disinfection of drinking water from surface and ground water sources. The use of lead-containing plumbing materials in public water systems and private drinking water systems that connect to public supplies was outlawed.

The amendments also increased protection of ground water, a crucial source of drinking water. They gave Indian tribes the same status as States in seeking primary responsibility for drinking water and underground injection control programs.

The major responsibility for safe drinking water rests with the water supplier, the State, and ultimately with the consumer as a concerned citizen. To stay informed about changes in standards and regulations, consult the EPA toll free Safe Drinking Water Hotline at (800) 426-4791.

Household Well Water. Approximately 15 per cent of the American public receive their drinking water from individually owned and operated sources such as household wells, cisterns, and springs. As "private" sources, system owners are solely responsible for the quality of the water provided.

Although private water supplies or wells are not regulated under the Safe Drinking Water Act, many States have programs to help well owners to protect their water supply. This safety information is particularly important because private wells are more shallow than those used by public supplies. The shallower the well, the greater the potential for contamination.

Well Water Contaminants. *Coliform bacteria* are the primary contaminants found in private well water. Septic fields, due to their location, are often the source of such contamination from animal or human wastes.

Nitrates are the second most common type of contaminant of private well water. The presence of nitrates suggests that animal or human wastes or fertilizers used in agriculture are entering the well. Nitrates are of special concern to the health of infants and young children, and women of child-bearing age.

Lead and *radon* are two other contaminants of concern to private well owners. Lead infiltrates drinking water through the corrosion of plumbing materials. The sources of lead in drinking water include lead pipes, lead-based solder, and brass faucets used in household and distribution system plumbing.

Radon exists naturally underground. As a gas, it can enter homes in two ways. First, radon can seep through soil into cracks in household foundations. Second, it can seep through soil into well water. When well water is agitated at warm temperatures in the home, as in a shower or washing machine, radon is released into the air. Airborne radon has been linked to lung cancer. Consequently, it is a contaminant of concern to public health officials and house-holders.

Contamination of private wells by other chemical contaminants remains a potential problem.

The degree to which any well is vulnerable to contamination depends upon a variety of factors:

- Local geology.
- Depth to water table.
- Soil, water, and climate characteristics.
- Local land-use and agricultural activities.
- Home plumbing materials.

GROUP CONTAMINANTS

The groups of contaminants of public water supplies for which standards are set include microorganisms, inorganic and organic chemicals, radionuclides, and disinfection by-products.

Microorganisms. This group includes bacteria, viruses, and protozoa: *coliform* bacteria, *legionella* , and *heterotrophic* bacteria; *enteric viruses;* and *Giardia lamblia.*

Inorganic Chemicals. The metals in this group include arsenic, barium, cadmium, chromium, fluoride, lead, mercury, nitrate, selenium, and silver. Lead is of chief concern and will be discussed later in detail.

Synthetic Organics. These are man-made, carbon-containing chemicals, and the ones currently regulated as pesticides and herbicides. The list includes 2,4-D, lindane, methoxychlor, endrin, 2,4,5-TP, and toxaphene. This group is sometimes referred to as Synthetic Organic Chemicals or SOCs.

Volatile Organics. These are organic chemicals which readily volatilize, or travel from the water into the air. They are commonly referred to as the VOCs. Most of them are industrial chemicals. The list includes trichloroethylene, carbon tetrachloride, vinyl chloride, 1,2-dichloroethane, benzene, para-dichlorobenzene, 1,1-dichloroethylene, and 1,1,1-trichloroethane.

Radionuclides. These radioactive chemicals are naturally occurring. Small water supply systems regulate gross alpha particle activity, radium 226, and radium 228. Larger systems are required to sample for beta particle activity in addition.

Disinfection By-products. These are chemicals formed when a disinfectant such as chlorine is added to water that contains organic matter derived from decaying plant or animal material. Total Trihalomethanes or TTHMs are those currently regulated. The MCL standard only applies to systems that serve 10,000 or more people and apply a disinfectant, such as chlorine, to the water.

The EPA is constantly in the process of revising standards and creating new standards for additional contaminants as these are recognized. Lead is one contaminant of drinking water of particular concern, particularly as it may affect the health of infants and small children, and child-bearing women. The EPA has research and abatement programs designed to reduce lead exposures to the fullest extent possible.

LEAD IN OUR DRINKING WATER

The sources of lead in our environment, the toxic effects and their manifestations, the treatment, and the prevention of lead poisoning are discussed in Chapter 1. Compared to lead-based paint and urban soil and dust, drinking water generally contributes relatively low to moderate exposures to lead. However, it affects large numbers of the population, and more than double the numbers exposed to lead in paint or dust. Lead in drinking water contributes between 10 and 20 percent of total lead exposure in young children.

The estimated number of children under 6 years of age exposed to various lead sources are compared in Table 9-4.

TABLE 9-4. Numbers of Children Under Six Years Exposed and having Elevated Blood Lead Levels.

		Blood Lead > 10 mcg/dL	
Lead Source	***Children***	***Number***	***Percent***
Paint	12 million	2 million	17
Soil and Dust	12 million	unknown	-
Drinking Water	30 million	1 million	3

Adapted from the EPA Strategy for Reducing Lead Exposures, February 21, 1991.

Lead levels in the drinking water are likely to be highest under the following conditions:

- If the home or water system has lead pipes.
- If the home has copper pipes with lead solder, brass faucets, or brass fixtures, and
- If the home is less than five years old, or
- If the drinking water is soft, or
- If water sits in the pipes for many hours.

The use of lead in pipes and solder was banned in 1986, but the EPA enforcement of this ban is limited.

The problem is found in houses that are either very old or very new.

Plumbing installed before 1930 is most likely to contain lead. Lead was also used for the service connections, goose necks, and water meters that join residences to public water supplies. This practice ended only recently in some localities. Copper pipes have replaced lead pipes in most residential plumbing. However, the use of lead solder with copper pipes is widespread, and is the major cause of lead contamination of household water in the United States today.

Lead enters the water after the water has left the local treatment plant or private well. Corrosion, a reaction between the water and the lead pipes or solder is the most common cause. All kinds of water may be contaminated but "soft" water is more likely to facilitate corrosion than "hard" water.

Contrary to popular belief, the newer the home, the greater the risk of lead contamination. Lead levels in household water faucets decrease as a building ages. Mineral deposits form a coating on the inside of pipes, and this coating insulates the water from the solder and reduces the corrosion. *Buildings less than five years old may have the highest levels of lead in the drinking water!*

Water Lead Level Standards. Until this year, Federal standards limited the amount of lead in water to 50 parts per billion (ppb), measured at free-flowing taps. In the light of new health and exposure data, the EPA has recently tightened this standard to a 15 ppb first flush "Action Level" at the tap. The EPA also requires all large water supply systems to optimize corrosion control for lead.

If the level of lead in the household water is in the area of 15 ppb or higher, it is advisable to take measures that will reduce the lead level to safer amounts, especially if there are young children in the home. Tap water should not be used to prepare infant formula.

The EPA estimates that more than 40 million U.S. residents use water that contains lead in excess of 20 ppb, when care is not taken to discard the first-flush water obtained from the faucet. Steady exposure to 20 ppb in drinking water would contribute between 2.5 and 3.5 mcg/dL to a child's blood lead level.

It is estimated that the new EPA regulations will result in the average blood lead level of those children not exposed to paint or soil contamination hazards to fall from 5.3 to 4.7 mcg/dL. Approximately half a million children with hazardous levels will have their blood lead levels reduced below 10 mcg/dL, and lead exposure will be minimized for millions of Americans.

MEASURES TO REDUCE LEAD IN WATER

- Refrain from drinking water that has been in contact with the plumbing for more than six hours. "Flush" the cold water faucet until the water is as cold as possible.
- Never cook with or consume water from the hot-water tap. Hot water dissolves more lead more quickly than cold water.
- Have your water tested for lead. Testing costs between $20 and $100. Testing is especially important

in high-rise buildings where flushing may not result in reduced levels of lead.

• Ask your public water supplier if the water is corrosive, and what steps are being taken to deal with the problem of lead contamination. Water mains containing lead pipes can be replaced, as well as those lead service connections that are the responsibility of the supplier.

• Calcium orthophosphate may be added to reservoirs to prevent lead from leaching into water.

• Well water can be treated to make it less corrosive. Calcite filters control corrosion and can be installed in the line between the water source and any lead service connections or lead-soldered pipes.

• Reverse osmosis devices and distillation units may be installed at the faucet to reduce the amount of lead in the water. These units can be expensive, and their effectiveness varies.

• Purchase bottled water for home and office consumption, if public water supplies are suspect. Bottled water is regulated by the FDA or by the State in which it is purchased, but controls are often fewer for bottled water than for public water supplies.

• Instruct plumbers to use only lead-free materials for repairs in the home or for new utilities.

• In a newly built home, remove all strainers from faucets and flush the water for at least 15 minutes to remove loose lead solder or flux debris from the plumbing.

• In homes where lead is a problem, water softeners should not be connected to pipes leading to taps supplying drinking water. A water softener may also contribute to the corrosiveness of the water and increase the potential for lead contamination.

• Note that carbon filters, sand filters, and cartridge filters do not remove lead from water and do not prevent corrosion.

GOVERNMENT AND A SAFE WATER SUPPLY

Drinking water is a precious resource and should not be taken for granted. Consumers should be concerned with Governmental measures to improve waste disposal practices and to clean up our environment. The emphasis on the environment in the recent presidential campaign, and the election of Senator Al Gore as Vice-President, should facilitate the passing of regulations that will ensure the safety of our nation's water supply.

In 1978, the Controller General of the United States issued a Report to the Congress which warned of the threat to health and the nation's water supply of unsound waste disposal practices. When water comes in contact with waste, it removes the soluble components and produces a grossly polluted liquid called *leachate.*

Leachate contains various decaying organics, bacteria, viruses, and toxic chemicals including heavy metals and carcinogens. Those areas of the country with the highest leachate contamination of water are also those with the largest concentrations of people, industry, and volumes of waste. These areas have millions of people obtaining water from public and private wells. EPA officials believe that land disposal sites pose a threat to public health through contamination of ground water and, eventually, of surface water supplies.

Contamination of Wells in Illinois. In Aurora, Illinois, seven domestic wells became polluted beyond use by leachate, within four years of opening a 22-acre landfill site. The contaminated water substantially exceeded drinking water standards and was particularly high in chlorides, organic acids, sulfate, sodium, and biological constituents. Families were without household water for 16 months. Their homes were finally tied into a public water supply system after legal action was initiated against the city and the disposal company.

Up to the time of the 1978 report to Congress, the relationship between waste disposal practices and groundwater was generally ignored by those responsible for disposing of waste. The States reviewed had only limited programs for monitoring disposal sites for evidence of contamination. Many sites not meeting State permit requirements remained in operation.

In passing the Resource Conservation and Recovery Act of 1976, Congress recognized that the problems of waste disposal are national in scope and require a broader Federal role. However, the improvements mandated were not accomplished within the legislative time frames. The EPA proposed that it would take several years merely to complete the open dump inventory, a key to improving the current practices.

Until this problem of waste disposal practices is rectified and our environmental groundwater supplies are made safer, the following steps can be taken to reduce the risks to our health of contaminated drinking water:

- Ensure that our water is treated to remove harmful contaminants.
- Test or monitor the purity of our water regularly to ensure its quality, and
- Develop an informed citizenry.

United States Environmental Protection Agency. Is Your Drinking Water Safe? September 1991.

Idem. Strategy For Reducing Lead Exposures. February 1991.

Idem. Citizen Monitoring: Recommendations to Household Well Users. April 1990.

Idem. The Safe Drinking Water Act. A pocket guide to the requirements for the operators of small water systems. 1990.

Idem. Lead and Your Drinking Water. April 1987.

United States Department of Commerce. Waste Disposal Practices: A Threat to Health and the Nation's Water Supply. Washington, DC, June 1978.

CHAPTER 10

PESTICIDE POISONS

Pesticide residues in our food and water have been accepted as almost unavoidable in light of the universal use of pesticides, herbicides, and fungicides in modern agriculture. The nutritional importance of pesticides has three aspects for consideration in regulatory measures to limit their use.

1) Protection of crops from pests and consequent increased production of food supplies.

2) Their effects on nutritive values of foods.

3) Health of the population.

GOVERNMENT CONTROL OF PESTICIDES IN FOODS

In the United States, the Environmental Protection Agency sets tolerance levels for the pesticide residues in raw agricultural products. Similar regulations are operative in other countries. National and international standards for pesticide residues have an influence on food trade, and lead to restrictions on consumption of some products from a State or country with higher maximum residue limits (MRL).

These restrictions and limitations are a concern to food buyers as well as the food producers, processors, and manufacturers of special products, such as baby foods and formulas. The levels of some pesticides, such as chlorinated hydrocarbons, in human milk may exceed the legal limits permitted in cows' milk. In fact, an analysis of human milk may be the most accurate measure of the extent of contamination of our environment by pesticide residues and other toxic chemicals.

Any decision to avoid feeding breast milk to infants or the ingestion of fruits and other foods known to accumulate pesticides to higher than expected levels must weigh the potential adverse effects of the residues against the nutritional benefits of the food.

The EPA and other national regulatory agencies establish acceptable levels of chemicals in foods that are based on toxicological data, the average daily intake of a food, and a safety limit. The risk-benefit ratio also involves the practical advantages of a particular chemical versus its known toxic effects.

Internationally, the World Health Organization (WHO) and the United Nations Food and Agriculture Organization (FAO) provide maximum acceptable daily intake levels for pesticides (WHO/FAO, 1972).

In addition to food, sources of drinking water may also be a reservoir for pesticide residues. Surface water contains chemicals from runoff, and ground water including wells may become contaminated.

Methods employed for the detection and analysis of pesticide residues are improving in sensitivity and specificity. They include gas-liquid chromatography, chemical ionization-mass spectrometry, and radioimmune assay. While individual pesticides rarely exceed the MRLs in food products, the dangers of interactions between multiple pesticides and potentiation of toxicity are not addressed by the existing regulatory measures in force.

THE PESTICIDE DILEMMA

The use of pesticides such as DDT to eliminate insects which damaged crops was widespread until their harmful effects on the ecology was realized. DDT was banned in the United States in 1972, and the use of other toxic pesticides has been restricted since then. Research is needed to investigate ways to employ pesticides to facilitate crop production without causing harm to the environment and adverse effects on the health of people.

DDT is a synthetic compound which cannot be broken down to harmless, inactive chemicals by animals. It is **nonbiodegradable.** DDT is also fat soluble. It concentrates in the tissues of animals and is transferred along the food chain, killing fish, birds, and mammals. **Biological magnification** is the term used for this increased concentration of chemicals as they ascend the food chain from small to larger animals.

The consequences of the DDT fiasco were the partial extinction of the bald eagle and golden eagle, and interference with the reproductive behavior of the osprey, falcon, and pelican.

Some pesticides, such as parathion, malathion, and phosdrin, do not spread through food chains, but they kill not only insects but predators of pests, thus disturbing the natural control of pest populations. The use of pesticides can sometimes make the situation worse and lead to multiplication of the insects.

Adaptation and the evolution of genetically resistant strains of pests has posed a problem for agriculture and the necessity to look for alternative methods of pest control. Resistance to pesticides has required limitations on the frequency of spraying and variation in the types of chemicals employed.

New ways in applying pesticides as an alternative to aerial spraying are being investigated. If chemicals could be applied more directly to pests, the volume of pesticide required would be substantially reduced and the risk of harm to other organisms would be minimized. Pesticide contained in plastic capsules and buried in the soil is one alternative to the spraying method.

ALTERNATIVES TO PESTICIDES

Toxic pesticides are not the only solution to pest control. **Biological control** uses organisms to check the increase in populations of pests. Insects, spiders, frogs, and birds are the natural enemies of pests and must be preserved to retain a natural, balanced ecosystem. Predators of pests such as the ladybird and wasps have been introduced in some areas of the country to destroy insects invading citrus crops and gypsy moths.

Spores of bacteria have been applied to lettuce, cabbage, and other vegetables to control the larvae of Japanese beetles. Viruses have been used against the cotton worm and gypsy moth. The disadvantages of pest control by microorganisms are the slow rate of action and an effect limited to only one specific species.

Autocidal control limits the size of pest populations by irradiation and sterilization of male insects. The use of sterile male medflies together with malathion successfully controlled the spread of this pest in California.

Hormones can affect the rate of metamorphosis of insects and are being used to control the growth of fleas and mosquitoes. Pheromones are used to trap insects or confuse them when in search of mates. The bark beetle which carries the fungus causing Dutch elm disease is susceptible to pheromones.

Cultural control of pests involves crop rotation, the optimal timing of planting and harvesting, and genetic techniques using recombinant DNA to produce pest-resistant plants.

The complexity of pest control demands more than one approach. **Integrated pest management,** a system that employs a combination of techniques, including chemical, biological, and cultural controls, is likely to be most successful. This approach might answer the pesticide dilemma while preserving the natural balance of the ecosystem.

PESTICIDE EFFECTS ON NUTRIENTS

While the use of pesticides generally results in an increase in total food production, the profitable influence on quantity may be offset by adverse effects on quality. Pesticide residues in the soil have been found to modify the nutritive values of certain foods.

Vitamin contents of vegetables and fruits, especially ascorbic acid and carotene concentrations, are often decreased by pesticides. In one report, decreases in ascorbic acid and niacin content were observed in various varieties of cabbage after treatment with the insecticide, carbotox. In other studies, the application of lindane to carrots resulted in a 15-50 percent decrease in carotene content; parathion reduced the ascorbic acid content of oranges; heptachlor caused decreases in starch and ascorbic acid in potatoes; and maneb decreased ascorbic acid and sugars in black currants.

Several studies of herbicides used in wheat production have demonstrated changes in the concentrations of lipids, proteins, calcium, and iron. Although some of these studies have shown variable effects and occasionally, increases in certain nutrients, the evidence for adverse pesticide-induced alterations of nutritive values of crops and food is strong.

Research to identify and reverse the negative effects of pesticides on human nutrition and health should play an important role in food production in the future. Economical considerations and the need to combat hunger in third world countries have encouraged the widespread increase in pesticide use in agriculture. However, the potential hazards of pesticide residues in our food cannot be ignored.

MECHANISMS OF PESTICIDE TOXICITY

Pesticides may be absorbed by the inhalation route, the skin, or by ingestion. The oral route is of greatest concern, since pesticide residues in foods and beverages are unavoidable contaminants of our diet. Their effects may be acute or chronic and delayed.

Acute Effects. Pesticides with acute toxic effects include neurotoxins, cholinesterase inhibitors, chlorinated hydrocarbons, DDT and derivatives such as methoxychlor, pyrethroids, formamidines, nicotine, metabolic inhibitors, arsenicals, rotenoids, inorganic fluorides, fluoroacetate, phenols, cyanide, organotins, haloalkanes, and paraquat and diquat. Table 10-1 lists some of these pesticides and the mechanisms of their toxicity.

Anticholinesterase agents (anti-ChE) form a large group of agricultural insecticides. Prior to World War II, physostigmine (eserine), a reversible anti-ChE, was the main example. During World War II, the organophosphates were developed first as pesticides and later as chemical-warfare agents. Their extreme toxicity was due to an irreversible inactivation of acetylcholine, causing paralysis of the muscles of respiration. Over 50,000 organophosphorus compounds were synthesized and screened for insecticidal potency, and many were produced for commercial use. Examples of this class of pesticides include parathion, sarin, and a carbamate, sevin.

TABLE 10-1. Pesticides and Mechanisms of Acute Toxicity.

Pesticide	*Chemical*	*Mechanism*
Cholinesterase inhibitors	organophosphates, carbamates	acetylcholinesterase inhibition
Organochlorines cyclodienes	toxaphene, aldrin, chlordane, lindane	release excess acetyl -choline
DDT-type	chlorophenothane	on nerve membrane
Pyrthroids	pyrethrum	cns & nerve synapse
Formamidines	chlordimeform	cns amine agonist
Nicotine		acetylcholine agonist
Arsenicals	arsenite and -ate	on Krebs cycle
Rotenoids	rotenone	on electron transport
Fluorides	sodium fluoride	inhibit glycolysis
Fluoroacetate	rodenticides	on citric acid cycle
Phenols	dinitro-o-cresol	on phosphorylation
Cyanide	hydrogen cyanide	inhibits c-c oxidase
Organotins	acaricides	on phosphorylation
Haloalkanes	methyl bromide	on sulfhydryl group
Bipyridiliums	paraquat, diquat	peroxide formation

Historically, physostigmine is an alkaloid obtained from the Calabar bean, once used as an "ordeal poison" in witchcraft trials by natives of West Africa. The first therapeutic use of the drug was in 1877 in the treatment of glaucoma. It is remarkable that the synthesis of an organophosphorus compound was published in 1854, some 10 years prior to the isolation of physostigmine.

CHRONIC TOXIC EFFECTS

Chronic or delayed toxic effects of pesticides occur as a result of continuous or repeated exposures to subacute doses, and are particularly important in relation to our food and diet. They involve many body systems and may be linked to a number of health problems.

Neurotoxicity. Organophosphorus compounds can cause a delayed neurotoxicity, characterized by neuritis and paralysis, the result of degeneration of myelin and nerve axons. This syndrome received widespread attention when an organophosphate, an adulterant of Jamaica ginger, was discovered to be responsible for an outbreak of thousands of cases of paralysis in the United States during prohibition.

A mammalian tremor caused by chlordecone poisoning may be due to effects on biogenic amines, and the neurotoxicity of the rodenticide Vacor in humans has been related to the inhibition of norepinephrine. Methylmercury causes a severe nervous system disorder characterized by tremors, incoordination, and paralysis.

A relationship between Parkinson's disease and exposure to pesticide chemicals has been demonstrated in a recent study at the Department of Community Health Sciences, University of Calgary, Canada. Individuals with a history of agricultural work and the occupational use of herbicides or insecticides showed a significantly increased risk of developing the disease.

Mutagenic and Carcinogenic Effects. Some pesticides such as toxaphene are strongly mutagenic, adding to the speculation that dietary factors and pesticide residues can be responsible for 50 percent of reported human cancers. For example, PCBs have recently been implicated in breast cancer research. The chemicals and mechanisms responsible for mutagenicity are also carcinogenic.

However, the National Academy of Sciences (1982) has concluded that it seems unlikely that large numbers of mutagens remain to be discovered in common foods, with the exceptions of mutagens produced by cooking.

Heterocyclic amines produced by cooking foods are mutagenic and carcinogenic, but their concentration is low and their potential risk is not known. Heat-stable antimutagenic factors have been isolated from cooked ground beef and caramel, and heat-labile mutagen inhibitors occur in raw vegetables and fruits. A mixed diet of meats, vegetables, and fruits should provide sufficient antioxidants, peroxidases, and inorganic minerals to act as antimutagens and offset the carcinogenic effects of some cooked foods containing pesticides.

Teratogenic and Reproductive Effects. DDT and chlorinated hydrocarbons have effects on the development of the fetus, causing various abnormalities and abortions. Oestrogenic effects cause decreases in libido, mammary development, and milk production in animals. In humans, the concentrations are generally considered to be too small to exert such effects, but the potential has not been properly assessed.

Behavioral Effects. Studies of behavioral toxicology of pesticide residues are limited to animal experiments in which very low levels have caused decreased learning and memory, hyperactivity, and aggressive behavior. The possible effects of pesticides in human milk on an infant's behavior are worthy of investigation.

Berger S, Cwiek K. Nutritional importance of pesticides. In: Hathcock JN (ed). Nutritional Toxicology Vol II, New York, Academic Press, 1987.

Coats JR. Toxicology of pesticide residues in foods. In; Hathcock JN (ed). Nutritional Toxicology Vol II, New York, Academic Press, 1987.

Koelle GB. Anticholinesterase agents. In: Goodman LS, Gilman A (eds). The Pharmacological Basis of Therapeutics 5th ed. New York, Macmillan, 1975.

Semchuk KM, Love EJ, Lee RG. Parkinson's disease and exposure to agricultural work and pesticide chemicals. Neurology 42: 1328, 1992.

Stich HF (ed). Carcinogens and Mutagens in the Environment Vol 1, Boca Raton, Florida, CRC Press, 1982.

Wiswesser WJ (ed). Pesticide Index 5th Ed. College Park, Maryland, Entomological Society of America, 1976.

CHAPTER 11

ALCOHOLIC BEVERAGES

"We drink one another's health and spoil our own."

Jerome K. Jerome, 1859-1927.

Alcohol is perhaps the most frequent toxin consumed regularly and in relatively large quantities by humans. Enjoyed socially for their pleasing taste and mood-modifying effects, the harmful effects of alcoholic beverages on our health are often forgotten or ignored.

During pregnancy particularly, a heightened recognition of the dangers to the unborn fetus linked to only mild to moderate alcohol consumption by the mother requires constant emphasis. It is estimated that as many as 5 to 10 percent of pregnant women consume amounts of alcohol sufficient to place their fetuses at risk of various malformations and developmental retardation.

FETAL ALCOHOL SYNDROME

The adverse effects of alcohol on the fetus were alluded to by Aldous Huxley (1932), in his "Brave New World": "What can be the matter with the fellow?" he wondered, and, shaking his head, decided that the story about the alcohol having been put into the poor chap's blood-surrogate by mistake......when he was still an embryo in the bottle.....must be true. "That's why he's so stunted." "Touched his brain, I suppose."

In the past 20 years, several medical publications have drawn attention to a characteristic pattern of birth defects in children born to alcoholic mothers. The most striking features of this "fetal alcohol syndrome" (FAS) are prenatal and postnatal growth deficiencies, microcephaly, facial dysmorphisms, mental and motor retardation, and structural abnormalities of the brain, heart, the joints, genitalia, and skeleton.

In initial reports of the FAS, the majority of infants exhibiting the full syndrome had been born to mothers consuming more than two grams of alcohol per kg daily. A total daily intake of more than 80 g was correlated with the occurrence of the syndrome in one study. Infants of mothers who were more moderate in their drinking habits were affected less severely.

A recent study at the University of Pittsburgh has identified and emphasized the importance of exposure to alcohol early in the first trimester as a cause of intrauterine growth retardation and developmental abnormalities in newborn infants. The average daily alcohol consumption of mothers with babies exhibiting none, one, or multiple defects was 0.69, 0.85, and 1.28 drinks per day, respectively. This dose/effect correlation was significant. The time of greatest impact of drinking was in the early part of the first trimester.

Research at the Wayne State University School of Medicine, Detroit, has shown that hearing disorders are a frequent complication of FAS and probably contribute to the speech and language and learning disabilities commonly associated with the syndrome. As a cause of mental retardation, FAS is as prevalent as Down's syndrome.

Between 1973 and 1991, 216 children with FAS were evaluated for congenital heart defects at the Universitat Munster and the Universitats-Kinderklinik Tubingen, Germany. Ventricular and atrial septal defects and other malformations were diagnosed in 63 (29 percent).

Incidence and Mechanism. The incidence of the FAS ranges from 1/300 to 1/2000 live births, and from 30-40 percent among infants of alcoholic mothers. The mechanism has not been definitely determined. Undernutrition is common in the alcoholic, and deficiencies in vitamin A, folic acid, and zinc may contribute to the etiology of the syndrome.

Alcohol in pregnancy, even as so-called social drinking, has to be considered an essential and preventable factor of mental and motor retardation and developmental defects of the brain, heart, and other organs. Until its exact role is determined, complete abstinence from alcohol during pregnancy and even during lactation is recommended.

Alcohol and Breast-Feeding. The relation of maternal alcohol intake during breast feeding to the infant developmental level at one year of age was investigated in 400 infants examined at the University of Michigan, Ann Arbor, and the University of Washington, Seattle. Motor development, as measured by the Psychomotor Development Index, was significantly lower in infants exposed regularly to alcohol in breast milk. Mental development was unaffected.

Nursing mothers can no longer enjoy the customary glass of beer as a prescribed method for sedating a sleepless baby without risking a detrimental effect on the infant's development. The practice of offering the parents a complimentary dinner with champagne at the time of discharge from some maternity units will have to cease, or if continued, with moderation and caution.

Long-term Effects. General pediatric, neurologic, and psychiatric reevaluations in a University of Berlin study of 54 children with FAS at four years of age showed improvement in facial appearance, and fewer neurological abnormalities. Learning abilities were poor, and hyperactivity and distractibility continued to impede their educational potential.

Of the 11 children first to be diagnosed with the FAS syndrome, two had died, one was lost to follow-up, and eight continued to show growth deficiency and dysmorphic facial features. Four of the eight were of borderline intelligence, and the other four were severely handicapped intellectually and in need of complete supervision outside the home.

Although the infant with the FAS may be recognized easily, the older child may not be as distinctive in appearance, making diagnosis more difficult.

EFFECTS OF ALCOHOL ON NUTRITION

Alcohol is a ready source of energy that is utilized more rapidly than most foods because it is absorbed quickly from the gastrointestinal tract and requires no digestion. When one gram of ethanol (ethyl alcohol) is metabolized in the body, 7.1 calories of energy are released.

Beer contains approximately 500 calories per liter, half of which is provided by its protein and carbohydrate content. In contrast, distilled spirits contain no additional foodstuffs and no vitamins, and their calories are derived purely from alcohol. A person who drinks 20 ounces of an 86-proof alcoholic beverage consumes about 1500 "empty" calories, because ethanol is lacking in significant quantities of protein, vitamins, and minerals. The intake of other foods decreases, and daily nutrient ingestion becomes grossly imbalanced.

Alcohol abuse leads to **primary malnutrition,** a deficient intake, and **secondary malnutrition,** a deficient nutrient utilization. Secondary effects on nutrition are caused by ethanol-induced gastro-intestinal damage, malabsorption of food, and energy wastage with loss of weight. The adverse effects of ethanol on the liver and other organs are also involved.

Mineral Metabolism. Metabolic balance studies of the effects of ethanol on mineral metabolism in healthy, nonalcoholic volunteers showed a negative balance of zinc, magnesium, phosphorus, calcium, and potassium, while sodium was unaffected. Losses of minerals, and the lowered serum levels of magnesium and calcium, result from increased excretion in the urine and/or feces, and a redistribution of minerals in cells of the tissues. Symptoms that accompany ethanol withdrawal, particularly myoclonus, may be related to the decreased magnesium levels.

Wine had a lesser effect on mineral excretion, and the balance of zinc was increased. Constituents in wine other than ethanol provide some protection of mineral metabolism.

Vitamin Metabolism. In alcoholics, a lowered serum folate level is the most prevalent vitamin deficiency, followed by low levels of thiamine and vitamin B_6. The incidence of low plasma pyridoxal phosphate (B_6) is more than 80 percent in patients with alcoholic cirrhosis of the liver and about 50 percent in alcoholics with normal liver histology.

Pyridoxine deficiency may underlie the occurrence of hallucinations and seizures during ethanol withdrawal, and thiamine deficiency is important in the complications of alcoholic polyneuropathy and Wernicke-Korsakoff syndrome.

Protein and Amino Acid Metabolism. Plasma levels of gamma-amino-n-butyric acid (GABA) and leucine are indices of chronic alcoholism. Carnitine deficiency is present in at least one third of alcoholics with liver cirrhosis.

Ethanol diminishes the uptake of certain amino acids by the brain, impairing the synthesis of neurotransmitter substances. Alteration in GABA levels following ethanol withdrawal is related to the occurrence of seizures.

Endocrine Effects. Feminizing signs, including breast enlargement and sterility, in male alcoholics are associated with hypoandrogenization. Alcohol-induced feminism is related to direct effects of ethanol on the testis, pituitary suppression, and to changes in hormonal balance produced by liver cirrhosis. The resultant decrease in the amount of testosterone leads to a failure of sperm production. An increase in estrogen accompanies the decrease in testosterone.

Shakespeare's comments in *Macbeth* on alcohol and sexual function are appropriate: In response to Macduff's question, *What three things does drink especially provoke* ? Porter answers:

> *Marry, sir, nose-painting, sleep, and urine.*
> *Lechery, sir, it provokes, and unprovokes;*
> *it provokes the desire, but it takes away the*
> *performance....*

ACUTE ALCOHOL INTOXICATION

Depression of the central nervous system is the principal manifestation of ethanol poisoning. Symptoms may be graded according to the blood alcohol concentration.

Mild (blood alcohol 0.05-0.15%; 0.5-1.5 mg/ml) - Levels above these limits are legal evidence of intoxication in most States. In Illinois, the legal limit is 0.1%. These concentrations can cause mild motor incoordination and a slowed reaction time. About 25 percent of individuals in this group have clinical signs of intoxication.

Moderate (blood alcohol 0.15-0.3%; 1.5-3 mg/ml) - Visual blurring, motor incoordination, slowed reaction time, and slurred speech are clinical manifestations of moderate degrees of intoxication recognized in 50 to 95 percent of this group.

Severe (blood alcohol 0.3-0.5%; 3-5 mg/ml) - These concentrations cause double vision, marked ataxia, stupor, and convulsions. Severe hypoglycemia and hypothermia are associated with occasional fatalities.

Comatose stage (blood alcohol >0.5%; >5 mg/ml) - Patients intoxicated to this degree are unconscious, their respirations are slow and shallow, reflexes and sensations are depressed, and fatalities are frequent.

CHRONIC ALCOHOL INTOXICATION

The consequences of chronic alcoholism are both medical and psychosocial. Factors such as dietary and nutritional deficiencies and liver dysfunction, which accompany alcohol abuse, may be responsible for some of the syndromes linked with chronic alcohol ingestion.

Gastrointestinal. Cirrhosis of the liver is the principal hazard to health caused by chronic alcoholism. Pancreatitis, and cancer of the oropharynx, esophagus, and liver are also related. Loss of appetite, gastroenteritis, and diarrhea lead to loss of weight and nutritional deficiencies.

Cardiovascular. Hypertension, cardio-myopathy, and heart irregularities are common complications, sometimes leading to stroke or sudden death.

Neuropsychiatric. Up to 50 percent of individuals diagnosed as alcoholics have been found to have signs of organic brain damage at autopsy. Syndromes of neuropsychiatric involvement include Wernicke-Korsakoff psychosis, cerebellar ataxia and degeneration, and polyneuritis.

Wernicke-Korsakoff Psychosis. In 1881, Wernicke described a syndrome characterized by the sudden onset of paralysis of eye movements, ataxic gait, and disturbed state of consciousness. Two of Wernicke's patients were chronic alcoholics and one was a young woman with persistent vomiting secondary to sulfuric acid ingestion.

The vast majority of cases of Wernicke's encephalopathy have been associated with chronic alcoholism, but isolated cases have been reported in nonalcoholic patients with vomiting in pregnancy and even in infants with nutritional deficiencies. At autopsy, the hemorrhagic lesions are concentrated in the hypothalamus of the brain, in the region of the third ventricle.

Symptoms and signs of polyneuritis and the memory and mental deficits of Korsakoff's psychosis are present in more than 50 percent of the cases. Many of the symptoms of Wernicke's disease, particularly the gaze palsies, improve dramatically after administration of thiamine, but the mental symptoms associated with Korsakoff's psychosis are not benefited.

Therapy includes withdrawal of alcohol, high caloric, vitamin B supplemented diet, and thiamine administered intravenously in large doses.

Delirium Tremens. An acute alcoholic mania may develop within 24 to 96 hours after cessation of a prolonged bout of steady drinking. Symptoms include uncontrollable fear, sleeplessness, tremulousness, restlessness, hallucinations, delirium, and convulsions.

Social Disorders. Family and child abuse, unemployment, suicide, accidental death, and even homicide may be related to chronic alcoholism. Traffic fatalities, falls, fires, suicides, illness, and domestic disputes, as consequences of alcoholism, have claimed from 50,000 to 200,000 lives a year, by one estimate. A report by the National Institute on Alcohol Abuse and Alcoholism in 1981 found that approximately 50 percent of drivers in fatal automobile accidents had been drinking before the accident.

Drinking while driving is particularly hazardous in persons with epilepsy, whose seizure control would be compromised by alcohol. Fortunately, the majority of epileptics are well aware of the consequences of alcohol abuse, and those permitted to drive an automobile usually demonstrate a responsible attitude toward their own safety and that of others.

Help for the chronic alcoholic patient and prevention of these complications may be obtained from Alcoholics Anonymous, for those who genuinely desire to receive treatment.

CHEMICALS IN ALCOHOLIC BEVERAGES

Allergies, headaches, and other hypersensitivity reactions to alcoholic beverages occur in certain susceptible individuals. The responsible agents are independent of the alcohol content of the liquor.

A long list of additives has been published, and many of the chemicals are potential toxins, capable of causing health problems. The majority of the reactions are not severe, but some are serious and may result in death. Unfortunately, the governmental regulations regarding labelling of foods and drugs does not apply to beers, wines, and liquors. A person with a serious allergy and asthmatic tendency could develop respiratory symptoms with fatal consequences if certain allergens were ingested unwittingly.

Beer Additives. Chemicals used in the brewing of beer include enzymes, clarifying agents, foam-stabilizers, antioxidants, artificial flavors, artificial coloring agents, and antimicrobial preservatives. The chemicals most likely to provoke allergic reactions are the antioxidants, especially the metabisulfites, and the artificial dye, FD&C Yellow No. 5. The FDA requires that Yellow No. 5 be declared specifically on all foods, but not including alcoholic beverages, which are not regulated by the FDA.

Apart from the chemical additives, the malt, rice, barley, or corn used in the brewing process may cause reactions in some allergic individuals. A knowledge of the exact ingredients of the beverage would save the susceptible consumer unnecessary discomfort and risk of injury.

Chemicals in Wine. Of the 80 or more additives permitted in wine making, sulfur dioxide or potassium metabisulfite is the one of greatest concern to the asthmatic and specialists in public health. Symptoms of an adverse reaction to sulfite include wheezing, tightness of the chest, breathing difficulty, and sometimes loss of consciousness. In very severe cases, the bisulfite may cause life-threatening anaphylactic shock and even death.

Winemakers use sulfur dioxide to kill bacteria on the grapes, to halt fermentation, and as a preservative. Using organically grown grapes, Californian winemakers have recently avoided the contamination of their product with insecticides and fertilizers, but sulfites are still included, particularly in the white wines.

Additives in Liquor. Of all alcoholic beverages, distilled spirits should be the safest for the consumer with allergies. Moonshine distilled in old automobile radiators has caused lead poisoning, and homemade whiskey contaminated with methyl alcohol has resulted in blindness.

Nitrosamines, a carcinogenic hazard in some beers and whiskeys, have largely been removed by changing the treatment of the barley. Distillation prevents contamination with most chemicals, but some are added to enhance color and flavor. Liqueurs especially contain additives such as caramel to add a brown color, non-dairy creamer as a substitute for real cream or "creme," and synthetic dyes to simulate real fruit, notably cherry and grape. Dyes with suspected carcinogenic properties in animal studies have been banned.

AVOIDANCE OF ALCOHOL RELATED ILLNESS

- Don't drink while pregnant or breast feeding.
- Don't drink while driving.
- Don't overindulge, acutely or chronically.
- Do maintain a healthy level of nutrition.

- Do take vitamin supplements, especially B vitamins, if a regular imbiber.
- Do avoid beers and wines, if allergic to sulfites and dyes.

Church MW, Gerkin KP. Hearing disorders in children with fetal alcohol syndrome: findings from case reports. Pediatrics 82: 147, 1988.

Day NL et al. Prenatal exposure to alcohol: Effect on infant growth and morphological characteristics. Pediatrics 84: 536, 1989.

Li T-K, Schenker S, Lumeng L. Alcohol and Nutrition. Research Monograph 2. Washington, DC, US Public Health Service, NIAAA, 1977.

Lipske M (Ed). Chemical Additives in Alcoholic Beverages. Washington, DC, CSPI Books, 1982.

Little RE et al. Maternal alcohol use during breast-feeding and infant mental and motor development at one year. N Engl J Med 321: 425, 1989.

Loser H, Pfefferkorn JR, Themann H. Alcohol in pregnancy and toxic heart damage in the child. Klin Padiatr 204: 335, 1992.

Millichap JG (Ed). Progress in Pediatric Neurology. Chicago, PNB Publishers, 1991.

Ritchie JM. The aliphatic alcohols. In: Goodman LS, Gilman A (Eds). The Pharmacological Basis of Therapeutics. 5th Ed. New York, Macmillan Publishing Co, 1975.

Sear MD, Norman MG. Two cases of Wernicke's encephalopathy in children: An underdiagnosed complication of poor nutrition. Ann Neurol 24: 85, 1988.

Seitz HK, Simanowski UA. Metabolic and nutritional effects of ethanol. In: Hathcock JN (Ed). Nutritional Toxicology, Vol II. New York, Academic Press, 1987.

Spohr H-L, Steinhausen H-Chr. Follow-up studies of children with fetal alcohol syndrome. Neuropediatrics 18: 13, 1987.

Victor M, Adams RD. Principles of Neurology. New York, McGraw Hill, 1989.

Wurtman RJ, Wurtman JJ (Eds).Nutrition and the Brain. Vol 4. Toxic Effects of Food Constituents on the Brain. New York, Raven Press, 1979.

CHAPTER 12

CAFFEINE TOXICITY

***"'Tis pity wine should be so deleterious,
For tea and coffee leave us much more
serious." Lord Byron, Don Juan***

Caffeine, theophylline, and theobromine are closely related xanthine alkaloids that occur in plants in different parts of the world. *Coffee* is a water extract of the seeds of *Coffea arabica,* containing caffeine. *Tea* is brewed from the leaves of *Thea sinensis* which contain caffeine and theophylline. *Cocoa,* obtained from the seeds of *Theobroma cacao,* contains caffeine and theobromine. *Mate,* a South American drink, contains caffeine. Caffeine-containing *Cola* soft drinks are prepared with the nuts of the tree, *Cola acuminata.*

Caffeine has stimulant effects on the central nervous system that account for much of the popularity of coffee, tea, and cola beverages. However, it can also cause adverse effects, including insomnia, restlessness, nervousness, and impaired performance on some tasks requiring fine motor coordination and timing. Of greater significance, but an issue less well defined, the possible effects of caffeine on fetal development are a concern. In addition, the pharmacological actions of caffeine affect the cardiovascular system, gastric secretion, intestinal motility, and urinary output, with harmful potential consequences when large amounts are consumed.

In limited or moderate quantities, coffee appears to be safe for the general adult population. In certain individuals and situations, however, coffee and other caffeine-containing beverages are best avoided.

HISTORY OF COFFEE

Kaffa, a province in Ethiopia, is reputed to be the birthplace of coffee. The original name is reflected by the words adopted for coffee in various languages: Chinese, *kai-fey;* Danish, *kaffe;* French, *cafe';* German, *Kaffee;* Italian, *caffe`;* Japanese, *kehi;* Polish, *kawa;* Russian, *kophe;* Turkish, *kahveh.*

The history of coffee is rich in legend, dating back to AD 850. One of the tales that surrounds the discovery of coffee concerns a goatherd named Kaldi who was bewildered by the strange behavior of his flock. Kaldi ate the berries of the bush on which the goats were feeding and was overjoyed at the feeling of exhilaration that he experienced.

The stimulating effect of coffee was used by some Muslims to sustain them through their long religious service. It was prohibited by the Koran because the strictly orthodox section of the priesthood claimed that coffee was an intoxicating beverage. Despite the severe penalties threatened for consumers, coffee drinking spread rapidly among Arabian Muslims, and its growth and use became ubiquitous in Arabia.

Coffee was introduced into Europe in the 16th and 17th centuries. It gained popularity as a beverage initially in London. The first London coffeehouse was established in 1652 at St Michael's Alley in Cornhill, and the first license to sell coffee in the United States was issued to a Dorothy Jones of Boston in 1670. In the 1960s, the US was consuming about 50 percent and Brazil was producing about 50 percent of the world's coffee crop.

It has been estimated that more than a billion kilograms of coffee are consumed annually in the United States alone. The popularity of the drink is related to its stimulant properties, aroma, and taste. The recent burgeoning of newly opened coffee houses throughout America attests to a growing demand for this form of stimulation or method of socialization.

Tea is the national drink of the United Kingdom, and its popularity has increased in the United States in the last decade. Cola-flavored soft drinks are a source of caffeine for Americans of all ages, and their consumption is probably equal to or greater than that of other caffeinated beverages combined.

The relative caffeine content of coffee, tea, and cola drinks is shown in Table 12-1. Tea leaves have a higher caffeine content than coffee berries, but the beverages provide approximately equal amounts of caffeine per cup. Cola drinks are relatively weak in caffeine, containing only one-third the caffeine of coffee and tea. Decaffeinated coffee has 1-4 percent the amount of caffeine contained in a cup of coffee.

The process of decaffeinating coffee was developed in Germany about 1900, and was later improved in the United States. The green coffee is steamed and then soaked in a chlorinated organic solvent. The removal of one potentially toxic substance may be accompanied by the addition of another!

TABLE 12-1. Caffeine Content of Xanthine Beverages.

Beverage	*Caffeine Content*
Coffee (beans)	0.7 - 2.0 %
Tea (leaves)	2.0 %
Coffee (cup)	100 - 150 mg
Tea (cup)	100 - 150 mg
Cola (12 oz bottle)	35 - 55 mg
Decaff. Coffee (cup)	1 - 6 mg

From Goodman LS, Gilman A . 1975.

MEDICINAL PROPERTIES AND SIDE-EFFECTS

Caffeine and other xanthine drugs have diverse effects on various organs of the body and provide valuable therapeutic applications. Caffeine is utilized chiefly for its stimulant effect on the central nervous system. Theophylline preparations, mainly aminophylline, are used in the treatment of asthma to relieve bronchial spasm and relax the bronchial smooth muscle. Aminophylline is also employed for its stimulation of heart muscle in the treatment of acute congestive heart failure.

Central Nervous System. Caffeine excites the nervous system at all levels. The stimulant effect on the brain cortex results in a more rapid and clearer flow of thought, and drowsiness and fatigue are allayed. After a cup of coffee, one is capable of greater sustained intellectual effort and association of ideas. Reaction time is shorter and the appreciation of sensory stimuli is more acute. This heightened sensitivity, or hyperesthesia, of the skin, experienced with overindulgence of coffee, can be an unpleasant sensation, and one indication of toxic excess.

Motor activity is increased by caffeine. Coffee is provided in secretarial offices, sometimes with the compliments of the employer, because typists who drink coffee work faster and with fewer errors. Studies have shown, however, that recently learned skills requiring fine muscular coordination may be adversely affected by one or two cups of coffee or tea.

Excessively large doses of caffeine in animals may cause convulsions followed by depression or death, but in man, fatalities from such reactions are very rare. In persons with epilepsy, coffee and other caffeine-containing beverages are contraindicated or permitted in moderation.

Stimulation of the medulla may improve the respiration and circulation in patients suffering from barbiturate poisoning. Theophylline is much superior to caffeine in its effect on respiration.

Caffeine causes constriction of brain arterioles with an accompanying fall in cerebral blood flow. The striking relief of vascular headaches, including migraine, experienced by some patients after drinking coffee is probably related to the vasoconstriction of cerebral blood vessels. Excess coffee may have the opposite effect, precipitating headaches in migraineurs.

Cardiovascular System. After large doses of caffeine, the heart muscle is stimulated and the pulse rate increases. Eventually this stimulation becomes sufficient to induce cardiac irregularities, or arrhythmias, in persons who consume caffeine beverages to excess.

A positive correlation was found between levels of coffee and tea drinking and the incidence of ventricular extrasystole in a sample of middle-aged men. In subjects with a history of cardiac arrhythmia, premature beats occurred twice as often when more than nine cups of coffee per day were consumed compared to two cups or less per day. Patients with a history of cardiac dysrhythmia related to caffeine consumption had an increased incidence of mitral valve prolapse, a condition often associated with high catecholamine levels.

The potential danger of production of ventricular arrhythmias by caffeine in subjects with cardiovascular disease seems established although the clinical significance is uncertain. The recommendation to those at risk for arrhythmias that they limit their intake of caffeine seems reasonable.

Coronary Heart Disease. Epidemiological studies that proposed a connection between coffee intake and coronary heart disease were later discovered to involve the smoking habits of the subjects as the more likely cause. An investigation in Norway, however, did reveal a correlation between coffee and levels of serum cholesterol which was significant when smoking and other risk factors were considered. Substantial increases in cholesterol levels have been demonstrated only in relation to doses of caffeine far larger than dietary intakes, and an increased incidence of atherosclerosis attributable to caffeine has not been found at any dosage.

Caffeine dilates the blood vessels of the heart, lungs, and systemic organs, causing an increase in cardiac output by a direct effect on the muscle within the artery walls. The use of caffeine in the treatment of coronary insufficiency is controversial and outdated. Coronary blood flow to the heart is increased but the work of the heart muscle and demand for oxygen are also increased. The effect of caffeine on blood pressure is unpredictable, but a slight rise may be expected in some individuals.

Smooth Muscle. Theophylline benefits asthmatics by relaxing the smooth muscle of the bronchi. It has also been employed for the relief of biliary colic, overcoming spasm of bile ducts caused by gall stones.

Skeletal Muscle. Caffeine has been found to increase the capacity for manual labor, and enhances the performance in long-term exercise such as cross-country skiing or marathon running. A direct effect on the muscle is a likely mechanism, since xanthines strengthen the contraction of isolated muscle elicited by electrical stimulation. The International Olympic

Committee has ruled that blood levels of caffeine must not exceed 15 mg/liter in participating athletes.

Diuretic Effect. All the xanthine drugs increase the production of urine. Theophylline is the most powerful xanthine diuretic, and caffeine is the least potent. An increase in renal blood flow and filtration rate, or a direct effect on the renal tubule are mechanisms proposed for the diuretic response experienced by coffee drinkers. Although this action of caffeine may be used therapeutically in some situations, in patients with a tendency to urinary incontinence the diuretic effects of coffee and tea can lead to embarrassment.

Gastric Secretion. Even moderate doses of caffeine ingested by coffee drinkers result in an increase of gastric secretion that is prolonged and abnormal. In animal studies, caffeine in small repeated doses causes stomach ulceration. Coffee, tea, and cola drinks may be factors in the cause of peptic ulcer and are best avoided in susceptible patients.

Teratogenesis. Administration of caffeine in doses of 50-100 mg/kg daily to pregnant mice resulted in an increase in the frequency of malformations in the offspring. Cleft palate and absent digits were the most common abnormalities induced. The interpretation of these findings must be treated cautiously, since studies in women who consumed caffeine in moderate quantities during pregnancy revealed no significant increase in the incidence of malformations in their infants. Women with a personal or family history of previous infant malformations would be prudent to limit their intake of caffeine-containing beverages during subsequent pregnancies, especially in the first trimester.

A delay in ossification of the bones of fetuses has been demonstrated in studies of pregnant rats fed caffeine at relatively low doses. The implications for advice to pregnant women or the older population with osteoporosis are unclear. Further investigations are required to determine if toxic levels of caffeine have a selective effect on calcium metabolism and bone development.

Hypertrophy of the hearts of rat pups has followed the daily administration of caffeine in doses of 10 mg/kg daily to the lactating dams and in the pup food. In contrast, no effect on heart size was observed in adult rats fed caffeine for as long as two years. Toxic effects of caffeine may be more apparent in the immature mammal, and the limitation of coffee, tea, and cola consumption in young children seems justified.

Fibrocystic Breast Disease. Abstention from caffeine consumption has been reported to relieve the symtoms of fibrocystic disease of the breast, Young women who develop this condition are generally advised to limit their intake of coffee and other caffeinated beverages. The dramatic effect observed in the initial study was not duplicated to the same degree in a subsequent series of patients, and some authorities are skeptical of the significance of the results. Fluctuation in cyst size will occur spontaneously, and assessment of treatment efficacy in disorders which may vary with time is difficult.

Behavioral Effects. The behavioral effects of caffeine are dependent on the condition of the subject tested and the nature of the task. A dose of caffeine that disrupts performance in the coffee abstainer may be restorative in the habitual user. One or two cups of coffee, containing 150-300 mg caffeine, in the morning produced nervousness in nonusers but alleviated these symptoms after a decaffeinated coffee had been substituted in individuals who were regular consumers.

A dose of 110 mg caffeine, equivalent to one cup of coffee, could slow completion of a figure discrimination task when first presented to undergraduates but facilitated performance when the task was learned previously. College students consuming up to eight cups of coffee daily reported low scores in psychological and somatic well-being and received relatively poor grades.

Hyperactive children are sometimes benefited by treatment with stimulant medications. A single limited study of coffee in 11 children with attention deficit hyperactivity disorder claimed a degree of success, but subsequent controlled trials of caffeine were without demonstrable significant effect. Coffee is not generally recommended for the management of behavior disorders in children, and its consumption by normal children is not encouraged.

Overconsumption of coffee may cause tremulousness, anxiety, irritation, agitation, sensory disturbances, and insomnia. Doses in excess of 500 mg caffeine have been cited as presenting a significant health risk, particularly in persons with psychiatric disorders. The DSM-III of the American Psychiatric Association (1987) defines caffeinism as follows:

CAFFEINE-INDUCED ORGANIC MENTAL DISORDER

305.90 Caffeine Intoxication

A. Recent consumption of caffeine, usually in excess of 250 mg.

B. At least five of the following signs:

(1) restlessness
(2) nervousness
(3) excitement
(4) insomnia
(5) flushed face
(6) diuresis
(7) gastrointestinal disturbance
(8) muscle twitching
(9) rambling flow of thought and speech
(10) tachycardia or cardiac arrhythmia
(11) periods of inexhaustibility
(12) psychomotor agitation

C. Not due to any physical or other mental disorder, such as Anxiety Disorder.

Obviously, the psychiatric profession regards caffeine as a potentially toxic drug capable of causing an organic psychiatric disorder, definable in diagnostic terms. The behavioral consequences of caffeine may be mistaken for symptoms of an anxiety disorder. Patients diagnosed with panic disorders were more susceptible to the "anxiety" effects of caffeine than mentally normal controls or those suffering from depression.

Clearly, caffeine-containing beverages may pose a hazard to certain psychiatric patients, and consumption of coffee should be limited, especially in those with anxiety and panic disorders. Indeed, some reports have suggested a self-limiting phenomenon and a voluntary avoidance of coffee in individuals who experience unpleasant effects.

Effects on Sleep. The effects of moderate doses of caffeine on sleep patterns in humans will vary depending on the timing, the frequency of usage, occasional or habitual, and the age of the individual. A cup of coffee 30 min prior to bedtime in young adults postponed the onset of sleep by about 20 min and decreased the total sleep time to the same extent. In older individuals and in persons suffering from insomnia, the bedtime intake of coffee may cause longer periods of wakefulness, and the inappropriate timing of dietary consumption of caffeine should be avoided.

Some degree of tolerance may develop to the sleep disorders caused by caffeine. The degree to which a person is stimulated by a given amount varies. Some persons have the ability to drink several cups of coffee in the evening and yet sleep soundly. Others with an exquisite sensitivity to caffeine develop symptoms of intoxication after only one cup. Decaffeinated coffee, containing 1-6 mg caffeine per cup, may be an acceptable substitute.

Overindulgence in caffeinated beverages can lead to a condition of **chronic intoxication**. Central nervous stimulation results in restlessness and insomnia. Cardiovascular stimulation is manifested by a rapid and irregular pulse. Gastrointestinal irritation is associated with heartburn and diarrhea. Urinary diuresis may aggravate a tendency to incontinence. Individuals who experience one or other of these side-effects should attempt a gradual reduction and avoidance of caffeine in their diet.

American Psychiatric Association: Diagnostic and Statistical Manual of Mental Disorders, 3rd ed, Revised. Washington DC, American Psychiatric Association, 1987.

Bergman J, Dews PB. Dietary caffeine and its toxicity. In: Hathcock JN (ed). Nutritional Toxicology Vol II, New York, Academic Press, 1987.

Encyclopaedia Britannica Vol 6. Coffee. Chicago, William Benton, 1963.

Gilliland K, Andress D. Ad lib caffeine consumption, symptoms of caffeinism, and academic performance. Am J Psych 138: 512, 1981.

Gould L et al. The cardiac effects of coffee. Angiology 24: 455, 1973.

Greden JF et al. Anxiety and depression associated with caffeinism among psychiatric inpatients. Am J Psych 135: 963, 1978.

James JE, Stirling KP. Caffeine: A survey of some of the known and suspected deleterious effects of habitual use. Br J Addict 78: 251, 1983.

Karacan I et al. Dose-related sleep disturbances induced by coffee and caffeine. Clin Pharmacol Ther 20: 682, 1976.

Klatsky AR et al. Coffee, tea and cholesterol. Am J Cardiol 55: 577, 1985.

Millichap JG. The Hyperactive Child with Minimal Brain Dysfunction. Chicago, Year Book Medical Publishers, 1975.

Minton JP et al. Response of fibrocystic disease to caffeine withdrawal and correlation of cyclic nucleotides with breast disease. Am J Obstet Gynecol 135: 157, 1979.

Ritchie JM. Central nervous system stimulants. The xanthines. In: Goodman LS, Gilman A (eds). The Pharmacological Basis of Therapeutics. 5th ed. New York, Macmillan Publishing, 1975.

Schnackenberg RC. Caffeine as a substitute for schedule II stimulants in hyperkinetic children. Amer J Psych 130: 796, 1973.

Wilson JG, Scott WJ. The teratogenic potential of caffeine in laboratory animals. In: Dews PB (ed). Caffeine. Berlin and New York, Springer-Verlag, 1984.

CHAPTER 13

FOOD ALLERGIES

"What is one man's food is another man's poison." ***Lucretius, 96 - 55 B.C.***

Food allergy refers to an adverse reaction to certain foods experienced by a small proportion of the population. The term is still used collectively by some physicians and many consumers to describe a group of clinical syndromes with diverse causes related to food intolerance. In recent years, **food sensitivity** has been accepted as more correctly representative of the broad range of individualistic reactions to foods. Pure food allergy is restricted to one category of food sensitivity caused by abnormal immunological reactions to a food or food constituent, usually a protein substance.

The subject of food sensitivity is controversial. It generates much public interest but an equal amount of medical skepticism. Skin tests for food allergy are unreliable, and elimination diets designed to avoid the offending allergen are troublesome and tedious. Specialists in allergy are frequently less than enthusiastic about the field. The medical acceptance of the diagnosis of food allergy has been hindered by the use of dubious techniques by some practitioners and the lack of validated laboratory tests.

In the past decade, several scientific reports using double-blind, statistically approved designs have been published. These studies have enhanced the credibility and confirmed the diagnosis of food sensitivity reactions as the explanation for a variety of clinical syndromes. True food allergy is common in infants and children with an estimated incidence of up to eight percent. In the overall population, the incidence is probably closer to one percent, although the perceived prevalence in some areas is much higher.

CLASSIFICATION

Food sensitivities are categorized into two main groups, primary and secondary. Table 13-1 shows the different types of food sensitivity reactions within these groups. The *primary group* includes a) the true food allergies, and b) the non-immunologic food intoxications and idiosyncrasies, sometimes called food intolerances. The *secondary group* of food sensitivities occur in association with various gastrointestinal illnesses and therapy with certain drugs.

TABLE 13-1. Classification of Primary Food Sensitivities.

PRIMARY FOOD SENSITIVITIES	
Immunological	*Non-Immunological*
Food Allergies	Allergy-like intoxications - scombroid fish poisoning
IgE mediated - cows' milk, eggs, peanuts, wheat	Anaphylactoid reactions
Non- IgE mediated, immune complex reaction	Metabolic - lactose, favism, celiac disease
Delayed-hypersensitivity reactions	Idiosyncratic reactions - sulfites, chocolate, dyes

FOOD ALLERGIES AND SENSITIVITIES

Food allergies are distinguished from other primary food sensitivities by the involvement of the immune system. Three types of allergic reaction can occur with foods: 1) IgE mediated, 2) non- IgE mediated, immune complex reactions, and 3) delayed hypersensitivity reactions.

IgE Mediated. Type I reactions are acute or immediate in onset and are due to the production of allergen-specific immunoglobulin E (IgE) in response to exposure to an allergenic food protein.

Common allergenic foods involved in type I food allergies are as follows:

- Cows' milk
- Eggs
- Peanuts
- Shellfish
- Soybeans
- Other legumes
- Wheat
- Fish

Cows' milk is the most common allergenic food in infants. Adults react especially to peanuts and shellfish. Casein and lactoglobulin are the allergens in cows' milk, and multiple allergenic proteins have been isolated from peanuts.

Two adolescent patients with anaphylactic reactions to the ingestion of mustard sauce were recently reported. Mediation by specific IgE to mustard was determined by skin prick tests and radioimmune assay, suggesting a type I true allergic mechanism. Hypersensitivity to mustard, a member of the Cruciferae family, is due to the protein contained in this vegetable. Reports of allergic reactions to mustard are rare.

Food allergies are often familial. Whereas peanut and fish allergies are frequently persistent, those to milk and eggs may be outgrown. In a recent report from the Netherlands, 88 infants studied for cows' milk protein intolerance (CMPI) by elimination challenge tests showed a gradual reduction in the number of positive reactors over a four year period. At ages 1, 2, 3, and 4 years, respectively, 15%, 22%, 51%, and 67% were no longer intolerant to cows' milk. Those infants with the highest initial levels of serum IgE were more likely to show persistence of cows' milk allergy at 4 years of age. The RAST blood test for IgE mediated food allergy had no predictive value for the development of tolerance with increasing age in these infants.

Symptoms of Food Allergies. The acute reactions involve the gastrointestinal tract, the skin, respiration, and larynx. Symptoms include nausea, vomiting, and diarrhea; urticaria, eczema, and angioedema; wheezing, asthma, and edema of the larynx; and headache, low blood pressure, and anaphylactoid shock.

Diagnosis. An IgE-mediated food allergy requires careful medical confirmation of the adverse reaction in close relation to the suspected food. Double-blind challenge tests (DBCTs) may be hazardous but are often essential to establish the role of a specific food. DBCTs may be contraindicated in patients who have reacted severely with anaphylactoid shock or laryngeal edema. The elimination diet followed by an open challenge is a more popular and practical test.

Once the suspected food has been identified, the diagnosis of IgE-mediated allergy is made with a skin test, the serum IgE determination, and the radio-allergosorbent test (RAST) on blood.

Non-IgE Mediated Reactions. These non-IgE mediated allergies are known as immune complex reactions. Typically, they develop within four to six hours of exposure to the offending food. The reaction that results is an inflammatory process initiated by the interaction of antigen with the immune antibodies and complement. The demonstration of tissue-bound immune complexes requires biopsy of the inflamed tissue.

Immune complex reactions occur in patients with cows' milk allergy and have been linked to cases of delayed intestinal inflammatory disease. IgG and IgM antibodies to various foods have been detected, but they do not correlate closely with symptoms. Specific avoidance diets are the only effective treatment.

Delayed-Hypersensitivity Reactions. The symptoms of this cellular hypersensitivity appear within 6-24 hours. They develop slowly, reach a peak at 48 hours, and subside after 72 hours. Unlike the other two types of food allergy, the reactions do not involve antibodies or complement. The interaction is between specific food antigen and sensitized T lymphocytes, generating soluble proteins called lymphokines.

Lymphokines and other cells released in the reaction result in histamine production and inflammatory changes. Delayed hypersensitivity reactions are sometimes involved in cows' milk allergies causing intestinal disease. The diagnosis is difficult and requires assays of lymphokines produced by lymphocytes in the blood. Treatment involves avoidance of the specific antigen in the diet.

Treatment of Food Allergies. Treatment includes 1) avoidance of the specific food allergen when clearly identified; 2) epinephrine or antihistamines for acute reactions, and 3) elimination diets to uncover offending foods responsible for chronic allergic reactions.

Food Avoidance. The avoidance of foods that provoke reactions is often difficult, and the inadvertent exposure is a frequent hazard. Meals eaten in restaurants are a common source of accidental consumption of the offending protein. Food labels must be scrutinized carefully but some are unreliable. Children sensitive to milk need to choose dairy-free products. So-called "non-dairy" products may be milk contaminated, however, and allergic reactions have been reported.

Food and Drug Administration proposed labeling reforms govern nutrient content and the identification of protein hydrolysates, including protein source, in the list of ingredients. The Canadian Restaurant and Food Service Association has introduced an allergy awareness program in which restaurants maintain lists of food ingredients for concerned customers.

An Expert Panel on Food Safety and Nutrition commissioned by the Institute of Food Technologists drew attention to the low degree of tolerance and exquisite sensitivity of some individuals with type I food allergies (1985). Some examples of a minimal exposure to an offending allergen sufficient to cause symptoms are as follows:

- Kissing lips of person eating offending food.
- Utensils contaminated by traces of food.
- Vapors from cooking of food.
- Opening packages of food.
- Breast milk transfer of allergen to infant.

Cross-reactivity can occur between related foods such as peanuts and soybeans, shrimp and crab, or cows' milk and goats' milk. Even"hypo-allergenic" foods used as substitutes are suspect, since allergies can develop to the substitute ingredients. For example, reactions sometimes occur to soybeans and goats' milk that are used as alternatives to cows' milk.

Breast-feeding, often advocated to prevent food allergies in infants, is not invariably successful. Allergies have been reported while the infant is on a strict breast milk regimen, or on the first exposure to a specific food at the time of weaning. Sensitization is caused by transmission of the food allergen in the breast milk.

Epinephrine Treatment. Children and adults with a history of anaphylactic sensitivity to food must be taught the importance of emergency kits containing epinephrine. Epinephrine is available commercially in spring-loaded self-injectable syringes. The failure to recognize the severity of these reactions and to administer epinephrine promptly increases the risk of a fatal outcome.

In a report from the Division of Pediatric Allergy and Immunology, John Hopkins University School of Medicine, August 1992, six fatal and seven near-fatal cases of food-induced anaphylaxis were encountered in children and adolescents in a 14-month period. Twelve had suffered from asthma that was well controlled with medications. All had known food allergies, but had unknowingly ingested the foods responsible for the reactions. Candy, cookies, and pastry were the sources of hidden allergens. The offending foods were peanuts (four patients), nuts (six patients), milk (two patients), and eggs (one patient). Nearly all the patients had had previous anaphylactic reactions to the same food.

A delay in the administration of epinephrine was associated with a fatal outcome. Five of the six fatalities occurred in schools or public places, whereas all the nonfatal reactions were in private homes where emergency treatment with epinephrine was available.

The American Academy of Pediatrics Committee on School Health has recommended that schools be equipped to treat anaphylaxis in children. Many states do not permit nonmedical personnel to administer epinephrine, and some state and local medical organizations have opposed legislation to certify laypersons to perform the injections.

Anaphylactic sensitivity to food in children is a difficult management problem for physician, parents, and teachers. The need to protect the child by food restrictions and elimination of allergens from the home must be balanced by the need to permit the child independence and self-esteem. Teachers must counsel classmates regarding the nature of the problem and the seriousness of accidental or intentional exposure to the allergen. Children have been known to test the allergic reaction by hiding the incriminating food in a child's lunch! Educational assistance may be obtained from the *Food Allergy Network* , 4744 Holly Ave., Fairfax, VA 22030, the *Asthma and Allergy Foundation of America,* 1125 15th St., NW, Suite 502, Washington, DC 20005, and other support groups.

Elimination Diets and Challenge. When chronic or multiple food allergies are suspected, an elimination diet that removes all but a few sensitizing food antigens is sometimes recommended. The complete omission of all possible food antigens would be impractical.

The diet consists of a small number of safe foods which have rarely produced reactions. Examples of hypoallergenic foods include lamb, potato, tapioca, carrots, peas, and pears. Foods excluded and most commonly found to be allergenic are cows' milk, cheese, eggs, wheat cereals, chocolate, nuts, and citrus fruits. In addition, food additives and salicylates are omitted.

If symptoms are relieved for a 10-day period, the omitted foods are reintroduced to the diet sequentially at weekly or shorter intervals. A genuine reaction to the challenge is usually obvious, and the offending food is then withdrawn.

Elimination diets are tedious but frequently successful, if parent and physician are compliant and enthusiastic. Allergists are often willing to use this technique only in the IgE-mediated food allergies, which account for a small proportion of cases of food sensitivity. Since the symptoms of food sensitivity can affect many organ systems, physicians from several different specialties may be involved. Some may be sufficiently interested to supervise the elimination diet themselves, whereas others may choose to consult a cooperative allergist. The services of a dietician are important, to ensure that the nutritional content of the diet is adequate.

Food Sensitive Disorders. In addition to the readily recognizable true food allergies with acute and subacute onset, food hypersensitivity can underlie various chronic and recurrent medical disorders. Double-blind, controlled studies involving dietary modification in patients with migraine, irritable bowel syndrome, Crohn's disease, and celiac disease have demonstrated that specific food sensitivity may play a significant role in the cause of these disorders. Elimination diets should be considered in the treatment of intractable cases of the above conditions, when alternative, more simple remedies have failed.

Other disorders in which the relationship to food sensitivity is less clear include asthma, eczema, rheumatoid arthritis, hyperactive behavior, and nocturnal enuresis. These disorders are frequently incapacitating or troublesome, and traditional forms of treatment are less than satisfactory. Despite the variable success rate with elimination diets in this group of disorders, a trial of dietary modification is warranted in patients with symptoms found resistant to alternative therapies.

NONIMMUNOLOGIC FOOD SENSITIVITIES

A wide variety of mechanisms can account for diseases associated with food sensitivities that fall outside the category of true food allergies. A joint report of the Royal College of Physicians and the British Nutrition Society classified these non-IgE mediated food sensitivities into two main groups:

- Drug reactions, e.g. caffeine, salicylates, dyes;
- Partial enzyme deficiencies, e.g. lactase.

Idiosyncratic Reactions. A reaction to a drug or chemical additive in food is sometimes called an idiosyncrasy, food intolerance, or an abnormal susceptibility peculiar to the individual. The mechanism or mechanisms of these adverse reactions to chemicals or certain ingredients in food are largely unexplained. A partial list of chemicals and food-related idiosyncratic reactions are shown in Table 13-2.

TABLE 13-2. Food-Related Idiosyncratic Reactions.

Food or Additive	*Reaction*
Chocolate (phenylethylamine)	Migraine headaches
Cheese (tyramine)	Migraine
Citrus fruits (octopamine)	Migraine
Caffeine withdrawal	Headaches
Salicylates in fruits, dyes	Urticaria, asthma, rhinitis
Sulfites in wine and salads	Asthma, anaphylaxis
Monosodium glutamate	Chinese restaurant syndrome
Food coloring additives	Hyperkinesis, enuresis

The role of the food ingredient in some of these reactions, such as sulfites and tartrazine dye in asthma, is well defined. Food colors and preservatives as the cause of hyperkinetic behavior and nocturnal enuresis is not so firmly established. Food additives are discussed in Chapter 5, and sulfites in alcoholic beverages in Chapter 11.

Sulfites. Foods containing the highest concentrations of sulfites include dried fruit, lemon juice, and salad bar lettuce (500-1200 ppm). Moderate concentrations are found in wine, lime juice, dried potatoes, grape juice, wine vinegar, gravies, maraschino cherries, and fresh shrimp (40-160 ppm). Smaller amounts occur in pickles, maple syrup, beer, pizza dough, beet sugar, fresh fruit salad, jams and jellies, cookies, grapes, and corn syrup (5-30 ppm).

The diagnosis of sulfite sensitivity requires a sulfite challenge test which should be performed in a hospital setting, where emergency epinephrine and resuscitation equipment are available. Asthmatics are often more sensitive to sulfites in acidic beverages than to sulfites in capsule challenges.

Treatment of sulfite sensitivity involves the avoidance of sulfited foods and beverages. A major problem is the individual variation in susceptibility or idiosyncrasy and the amount and type of sulfite expected to cause a reaction. Sulfites can bind to food components such as sugars, proteins, and vitamins, and bound forms of sulfite predominate in most foods. The reactivity of sulfite sensitive asthmatics to bound sulfite is probably less than that to free sulfite, as found in wines, beer and lettuce. Lettuce is an unusual food in that the 400 ppm or more of total sulfite remains in and on the surface of the leaves as free sulfite.

Sucrose reactivity. Sucrose as a factor in aggressive, hyperactive, and delinquent behaviors is a controversial food related reaction. Consumer groups have expressed concern that sugar intake may induce hyperactivity by leading to abnormal swings in the level of blood glucose in certain susceptible children. For each report condemning sucrose in the diet of school children, another negates the role of sugar as a cause of behavioral disorders. Even if confirmed, the mechanism of sucrose-related brain dysfunction is unclear and may not be due to hypoglycemia.

When a meal rich in sugar and other carbohydrates is eaten, the brain is stimulated to make more of a neurotransmitter substance, serotonin, a chemical that modifies nerve cell function. Serotonin in the brain has functions concerned with attention and motor activity. Notwithstanding the paucity of controlled studies, certain individuals do appear to have an idiosyncrasy to sucrose, and some concerned parents believe firmly in the benefits of limiting sugar intake in their hyperactive children.

Anaphylactoid Reactions. These food sensitivity reactions are caused by substances that induce the release of histamine from tissue mast cells without involvement of immunoglobulin E. The urticarial reaction that occurs in some individuals after eating strawberries is the best example of an anaphylactoid food sensitivity. Treatment involves the avoidance of the offending food.

Histamine-Scombroid Fish Poisoning. The allergy-like intoxication associated with the consumption of scombroid fish (tuna, mackerel, bonito) is caused by the histamine contained in the fish. This form of histamine poisoning differs from the anaphylactoid reactions because the histamine is exogenous and is ingested as a part of the food; it is not secreted endogenously in response to the food.

Histamine is formed in foods primarily as the result of spoiling and bacterial action. Scombroid fish are especially prone to form histamine during spoilage because they have high levels of the amino acid, histidine, a precursor of histamine in their muscle tissues.

Symptoms of Histamine Poisoning. These are similar to the symptoms observed with true food allergies. The most prevalent are a skin rash, urticaria, vomiting, and abdominal pain. The onset is usually rapid, within a few minutes to a few hours. The illness is short and often mild, symptoms remitting within hours.

Treatment. Antihistamines may be of value in the relief of discomfort. In prevention, raw fish should be refrigerated to avoid spoilage during storage. The consumption of raw fish such as tuna should be limited.

Lactose Intolerance. Lactose intolerance is caused by an inability to break down lactose in milk into galactose and glucose, sugars that can be absorbed in the intestine. Lactose cannot be absorbed unless it is first hydrolysed by the enzyme lactase into the monosaccharide sugars. Undigested lactose passes through the small intestine into the colon where bacteria break it down to form the gas, carbon dioxide, and water. This gas formation causes the symptoms and discomfort of lactose intolerance, consisting of abdominal pain, flatulence, and diarrhea.

Patients who suffer from lactose intolerance are mainly older. With increasing age, the enzyme lactase in the intestine decreases in concentration. The incidence also varies with race and ethnic origin. Whereas approximately 10 percent of Caucasians are affected, the incidence among Arabs, black Americans, Greeks, Jews, and Orientals has been estimated at 60-90 percent.

Treatment. A reduction in the amount of dairy products containing lactose in the diet is often sufficient to allay symptoms. Complete exclusion of milk intake is necessary in only a few patients. Lactose-hydrolyzed milk, and fermented dairy products such as yogurt and acidophilus milk are often tolerated as alternatives. Calcium supplements to prevent osteoporosis are advised in patients who need to limit their intake of milk.

Favism and *Celiac Disease* are additional examples of food sensitivity reactions due to specific enzyme deficiencies.

Favism. Fava beans are responsible for an acute hemolytic anemia that develops in susceptible individuals within 6-24 hours after the ingestion of the broad beans or the inhalation of the plant pollen. The deficiency of an enzyme G-6-PD in affected patients causes their red blood cells to be sensitive to damage from oxidant chemicals in the fava bean.

The enzyme G-6-PD deficiency is genetically determined and occurs primarily in individuals born in the Mediterranean area, the Middle East, and China, where fava beans are a staple in the diet. An assay of the enzyme activity in red blood cells is used in diagnosis. A deficiency is only of importance in populations that grow and eat fava beans.

Symptoms of favism include anemia, pallor, lassitude, nausea, abdominal pain, and fever. Jaundice and kidney failure are rare complications. The disease is usually self-limiting, and recovery is prompt and complete.

Celiac Disease. Samuel Gee, a physician at Saint Bartholomew's Hospital, London, wrote the first description of celiac disease in 1888, "On the Coeliac Affection." Gee described the disease as a chronic form of indigestion, occurring most commonly in children, and characterized by a diarrhea with pale loose stools, wasting of the limbs, and distension of the belly. He attributed the cause to a faulty diet and failure of digestion, and he found cows' milk and highly starchy food to be unfit.

In 1953, Dicke and colleagues published a report of a factor in wheat having a deleterious effect in cases of celiac disease. After fractionating wheat into its four main components, fiber, fat, starch, and protein, the *gliadin* fraction of the water-insoluble protein, *gluten,* in wheat was found to be the offending dietary factor in celiac disease. Gee's description of the clinical symptoms and signs of celiac disease survives as a classic report of the disorder, and his understanding of the cause was close to that subsequently uncovered. It is a sad reflection on medical science and the relative lack of governmental funding for research that 65 years were allowed to elapse between the first complete account of an incapacitating intestinal disorder and the discovery of a simple, dietary related cause and treatment!

Both celiac disease in children and idiopathic sprue in adults are related to dietary gluten. The term *gluten-sensitive enteropathy* is now preferred. The prevalence of the disease in the United States is about 1 in 3000, but in parts of Ireland, it affects 1 in every 300 individuals. The symptoms are typical of a malabsorption syndrome, dependent on an inherited trait. The lack of some enzyme necessary for the digestion of gluten is one likely hypothesis, but the underlying deficiency is unknown.

Seizures complicate celiac disease in some patients, and cerebral calcifications have been reported in CT imaging. The significance of the calcification is undetermined but the finding is sufficiently frequent to recommend tests for celiac disease in patients with epilepsy and brain calcifications. Unlike the diarrheal symptoms of celiac disease, the seizures are not responsive to a gluten-free diet.

Diagnosis. A biopsy of the jejunal intestine and an anti-gliadin antibody test provide a definitive diagnosis. Improvement following a gluten-free diet and a normal post-treatment biopsy will confirm the diagnosis.

Treatment. In principle, the dietary elimination of all foods containing gluten appears simple. This entails the avoidance of wheat, rye, barley, and oats and any food products made from these grains. In practice, the adherence to such avoidance diets is often difficult. Wheat flower is used in many of to-day's prepared foods, including ice-cream, and the elimination of cereals may not suffice. The development of grain that does not contain the gliadin has been proposed as a possible solution.

SECONDARY FOOD SENSITIVITIES

A preexisting illness or drug therapy may predispose a patient to food sensitivity reactions. Viral or bacterial gastroenteritis, and ulcerative colitis have preceded the onset of lactose intolerance and celiac disease. Histamine reactions due to ingestion of tuna fish have been reported in patients treated with isoniazid for tuberculosis. Reactions to tyramine-containing foods are enhanced in patients receiving drugs for depression.

Our awareness of dietary migraine and its chemical mechanism stems from the observation reported by Dr. Edda Hanington in the British Medical Journal, 1967, of the headache reaction to cheese eaten by patients treated with monoamine oxidase (MAO)-inhibitors. The enzyme MAO in normal individuals will metabolize tyramine, the migraine provoking chemical found in cheese and other foods. Dr. Hanington postulated that patients with dietary migraine were sensitive to tyramine-containing foods by virtue of a deficiency of MAO in their tissues and blood. Dietary tyramine is one of many stimuli that may trigger a headache in a person with migraine. Table 13-3 lists foods and beverages known to precipitate migraine.

TABLE 13-3. Partial List of Migraine-Precipitating Foods and Beverages.

- Aged or strong cheese
- Cured meats (hot dogs, bacon, ham, salami)
- Citrus fruits
- Chocolate, cocoa
- Nuts
- Ice cream, yogurt, sour cream
- Chinese food (monosodium glutamate)
- Pork, seafood, chicken livers, herring
- Canned figs, beans, tomatoes
- Coffee, tea, cola drinks
- Alcoholic beverages

Adapted from Millichap JG. Nutrition, Diet, and Your Child's Behavior. Springfield, Illinois, Charles C Thomas, 1986, and other sources.

The amine-containing foods most frequently cited as dietary triggers of migraine are cheese, especially aged, strong and cheddar varieties, chocolate, and citrus fruit. While tyramine is considered the principle offending chemical, other amines, including beta-phenylethylamine and histamine, have been identified in chocolate and red wine.

Sulfites in wine and beer, and nitrites in hot dogs are additional ingredients in foods and beverages that may trigger headaches. Fatty acids, primarily linoleic and oleic acids, have also been invoked in the mechanism of migraine attacks.

Studies at The Hospital For Sick Children, Great Ormond Street, London, involving children with migraine, have demonstrated that cows' milk, egg, and wheat cereals frequently provoke headaches in addition to amine rich foods such as chocolate, orange, and cheese. The intolerance to such a wide variety of foods supported an allergic mechanism for dietary migraine rather than a metabolic idiosyncrasy to tyramine and other chemicals. Of 88 patients treated with an "oligoantigenic diet," a regimen that eliminates the majority of sensitizing food antigens, 93 percent with severe frequent migraine were free of headaches.

When foods were reintroduced at intervals and in sequence, 90 percent of the patients who had responded to dietary therapy relapsed. Fifty-five different foods provoked headaches when reintroduced to the diets. Skin tests and immune globulin antibodies showed no correlation with the provoking and non-provoking foods in this group of patients. The food sensitivity reaction was not IgE mediated.

SUMMARY AND CONCLUSIONS

The classifications of food allergies or sensitivities on the basis of mechanisms are sometimes poorly defined, and many are undetermined. Food allergy mediated by allergen-specific immuno-globulin E (IgE) is responsible for only a proportion of food sensitivities. Idiosyncratic reactions to additives and various drugs and chemicals in food are probably more common than true food allergies.

Partial enzyme deficiency, such as lactose intolerance, could prove to be the most important cause of food sensitivity. Many chronic and degenerative diseases of unknown etiology may represent reactions to various food additives or ingredients in individuals lacking some protective enzyme. Further research in this area of food sensitivity has been proposed by some authorities.

The skepticism surrounding food allergy in the medical profession has discouraged many physicians from entering the field. Its rejection by the academic community has in turn restricted research and neglected medical student exposure. Dr Finn, Consultant in Allergy, at the Royal Liverpool Hospital, England, notes that, "A more liberal view by the academic community could lead to the opening up of an important area of clinical science." "Perhaps clinical allergists should widen their horizon from IgE reactions and accept responsibility for the management of food sensitivity in its broad sense."

By coincidence and almost in response to this criticism, two prestigious medical journals in the

United States, the Journal of Pediatrics and the Journal of the American Medical Association, have devoted current issues to the subject of food allergies. It is hoped that these timely publications will serve to emphasize the importance of the health risks of food sensitivities in some individuals and point the way for future research studies.

American Academy of Pediatrics Committee on School Health. Guidelines for urgent care in schools. Pediatrics 1990; 86:999.

Anderson JA, Sogn D. Adverse reactions to foods. American Academy of Allergy and Immunology Committee on Adverse Reactions to Foods, National Institute of Allergy and Infectious Diseases. NIH publication No. 84-2442. Washington DC. US Government Printing Office, 1984:4.

Bock SA. Adverse reactions to foods during the first three years of life. J Allergy Clin Immunol 1985; 75: 178.

Darlington LG, Ramsey NW, Mansfield JR. Placebo-controlled, blind study of dietary manipulation therapy in rheumatoid arthritis. Lancet 1986; 1: 236.

Dicke WK, Weijers HA, van der Kamer JH. Coeliac disease. II. The presence in wheat of a factor having a deleterious effect in cases of coeliac disease. Acta Paediat 1953; 42: 34.

Dusseldorp M, Katan MB. Headache caused by caffeine withdrawal among moderate coffee drinkers switched from ordinary to decaffeinated coffee: a 12 week double blind trial. BMJ 1990; 300: 1558.

Egger J, Carter CM, Wilson J, Turner MW, Soothill JF. Is migraine food allergy? A double blind controlled trial of oligo antigenic diet treatment. Lancet 1983; 2: 865.

Egger J et al. Controlled trial of hyposensitization in children with food induced hyperkinetic syndrome. Lancet 1992; 339: 1150.

Finn R. Food allergy-fact or fiction: a review. J R Coll Physicians 1992; 85: 560.

Food Intolerance and Food Aversion. A joint report of the Royal College of Physicians and the British Nutrition Foundation. J R Coll Physicians 1984; 18: 83.

Ferguson A. Food sensitivity or self-deception. N Engl J Med 1990; 323: 476.

Ferguson A. Definitions and diagnosis of food intolerance and food allergy: Consensus and controversy. J Pediatr Nov 1992; 121(Suppl): S7.

Gee S. On the coeliac affection. St Barts Hosp Reports 1888; 24: 17.

Gern JE, Yang E, Evrard HM, Sampson HA. Allergic reactions to milk-contaminated "nondairy" products. N Engl J Med 1991; 324: 976.

Institute of Food Technologists' Expert Panel on Food Safety and Nutrition. Food allergies and sensitivities. Food Technol 1985; 39: 65.

Jones VA et al. Food intolerance: a major factor in the pathogenesis of irritable bowel syndrome. Lancet 1982; 2: 1115.

Millichap JG. The Hyperactive Child with Minimal Brain Dysfunction. Chicago, Year Book Medical Publ, 1975.

Millichap JG. Nutrition, Diet, and Your Child's Behavior. Springfield, Illinois, Charles C Thomas, 1986.

Millichap JG. Food-induced hyperkinesis. Ped Neur Briefs 1992; 6: 63.

Monreal P, Botey J, Pena M et al. Mustard allergy. Two anaphylactic reactions to ingestion of mustard sauce. Ann Allergy 1992; 69: 317.

Sampson HA, McCaskill CC. Food hypersensitivity and atopic dermatitis: evaluation of 113 patients. J Paediatr 1982; 107: 669.

Sampson HA, Mendelson L, Rosen JP. Fatal and near-fatal anaphylactic reactions to food in children and adolescents. N Engl J Med 1992; 327: 380.

Sampson HA, Metcalfe DD. Food allergies. JAMA Nov 25 1992; 268: 2840.

Schrander JJP, Oudsen S, Forget PP, Kuijten RH. Follow up study of cow's milk protein intolerant infants. Eur J Pediatr 1992; 151: 783.

Schreiber RA, Walker WA. Food allergy: facts and fiction. Mayo Clin Proc 1989; 64: 1381.

Stern M, Walker WA. Food allergy and intolerance. Ped Clin N Amer 1985; 32: 471.

Taylor SL. Allergic and sensitivity reactions in food components. In: Hathcock JN (ed). Nutritional Toxicology Vol II, New York, Academic Press, 1987.

Warner JO. Food allergy in fully breast fed infants. Clin Allergy 1980; 10: 133.

Yunginger JW, Sweeney KG, Sturner WQ et al. Fatal food-induced anaphylaxis. JAMA 1988; 260: 1450.

CHAPTER 14

FOOD SAFETY CONTROLS

Potentially toxic substances may contaminate food in a variety of ways. Many originate in the environment from nuclear fall out and industrial wastes. Chemical residues of fertilizers, defoliants, and pesticides are added to vegetables and fruits intentionally during agricultural production, and occasionally they are consumed by accident when applied to grain. Mycotoxins contaminate stored foods whenever conditions of temperature and humidity are conducive to the growth of molds.

A list of potential food poison risks is shown in Table 14-1. In addition to environmental, agricultural, horticultural, and storage risks, the commercial processing of foods is a major source of contamination. Food packaging materials have health implications, and the domestic preparation and methods of cooling and storage of food are sources of concern. Finally, the consumer may expose himself or herself to risk by unwittingly overdosing with vitamins and minerals, or by ingesting foods containing allergens or chemicals that cause individual sensitivity reactions.

FOOD PROCESSING RISKS

During the commercial processing of food, the potential risks of contamination with chemicals and toxins are both intentional and unintentional. Food additives, preservatives, sweeteners, colorants, and flavoring agents are added by design. Heating or smoking may cause "pyrolysis," or decomposition of organic substances. Contaminants from machines and processing tanks include lubricants, metals, detergent cleaning agents, and thermal conductor PBBs. Botulinum and other bacterial toxins may form in low-acid canned foods and in honey. Cobalt chloride has been employed in the brewing of beer, with tragic consequences.

TABLE 14-1. Potential Food Risks and Their Origins.

Origin	*Food Poison Risk Factors*
Environmental	Nuclear, industrial wastes
Agricultural	Fertilizers, pesticides
Storage	Mycotoxins, fumigants
Processing	Additives, PBBs, bacterial toxins
Packing	Plasticizers
Cooking	Ceramics (lead), bacteria
Consumer	Megavitamins, allergens, enzyme lack

FOOD PACKAGING CONTROLS

Food packaging is important to protect foods against infestation and contamination as well as light, moisture and oxygen, which can cause decomposition. The packaging material is in intimate contact with the food for extended periods and sometimes, at elevated temperatures. Under such conditions, the migration of constituents of the packaging materials into the foods poses a hazard. Controls have been established to guard against the risk of toxic chemicals in packaging that might endanger the health of the consumer.

Regulatory agencies responsible for health protection have focused attention on the possible hazards of plastic-based food packaging materials. Traditional packaging, made from glass, steel, tinplate, paper, and paper-board, is relatively safe, but plastic trays for microwave cooking and plastic bottles for soft drinks and ketchups contain a variety of base polymers, antioxidants, colorants, and other additives.

In toxicology, food intake data are used to calculate the potential risk of ingestion of contaminants used as additives, pesticide residues, and those contained in packaging materials. The World Health Organization has a number of publications describing methods for estimating dietary exposure to chemical contaminants.

The chemical migrants from plastics of particular concern to health authorities are vinyl chloride polymers (PVC), acrylonitrile polymers (ABS), di(2-ethylhexyl) phthalate (DEPH), di(2-ethylhexyl) adipate (DEHA), and nitrosamines (NA). All have been found to cause cancer in animals and some in humans.

It may surprise consumers to realize the enormous potential for risk of intoxication from a multitude of migrant chemicals contained in plastic containers. It is equally reassuring to learn of the steps taken by the Food and Drug Administration, the Environmental Protection Agency, and other governmental authorities to protect the consumer from these hidden hazards. For example, enforced improvements in technology effected dramatic reductions in vinyl chloride levels in foods, and the use of acrylonitrile copolymer (ABS) bottles for packaging soft drinks and other beverages was banned by the FDA in 1977.

Acrylonitrile is an animal carcinogen and it concentrates in beverages and foods in significant concentrations during prolonged storage. A United Kingdom survey in 1982 showed that ABS levels in margarine tubs was 100 ppm. In the same year, Canada prohibited the sale of foods in packaging materials that contribute detectable amounts of acrylonitrile to foods.

In accordance with the World Health Organization Committee recommendations on Food Additives, the dietary exposures to vinyl chloride, acrylonitrile, and other packaging materials is now controlled in several countries. From a desire by trading countries to eliminate international barriers, several initiatives have been taken to control food packaging materials and their potential health risks.

As consumers, we have little or no control over potential food risks introduced via the environment, methods of agriculture, commercial processing, restaurants, or packaging materials. However, we can limit the risks of food poisoning by 1) care in the preparation and storage of food in the kitchen, 2) avoidance of overdoses of certain vitamins and minerals, and 3) reducing exposure to food allergens in susceptible individuals.

CONSUMER FOOD SAFETY CONTROLS

•To protect against lead, run the water until cold, before using for drinking or cooking.

•Avoid use of hot water tap for drinking, cooking, or mixing infant formula.

•Don't use pottery or cans to store foods or beverages.

•Don't store liquor in crystal decanters.

•To protect against PCB, mercury, DDT, and Dioxin, limit ingestion of fish caught in inland lakes and streams.

•Avoid excess doses of iron and vitamins A, D, B_6.

•Limit intake of aspartame in migraine or epilepsy patients and avoid in PKU children.

•Avoid additives, preservatives, and colorants in reactive hyperkinetic children.

•Avoid aflotoxins by discarding foods with mold growth or odor.

•Limit nitrates and nitrites by washing vegetables and fruits , limiting intake of hot dogs and salami, and checking well water for nitrate content.

•Protect against foodborne infections and toxins by avoidance of all raw meats, maintaining foods at $<10^oC$ during storage and at $10\text{-}50^oC$ while serving, and reheating inadequately cooled foods to 60°C before serving.

•If asthmatic or subject to other allergies, avoid sulfite-containing foods or beverages and other specific food allergens or additives.

The above list of avoidances and precautions for consumers to follow is incomplete. The suggestions are offered as generalizations. Each consumer is an individual, subject to a different set of environmental circumstances and a variable degree of reactivity to potential food poisons. The list should alert the consumer to the diversity of dietary risk factors and ways to avoid them. Consultation with a physician, dietician, or other professional may be necessary for individuals with specific food sensitivities and risks of exposure.

Ariens EJ, Simonis AM. General principles of nutritional toxicology. In: Hathcock JN (ed). Nutritional Toxicology Vol III, New York, Academic Press, 1989.

Kirkpatrick DC, Ripley RA, Pelletier MA. Food packaging materials: health implications. In: Hathcock JN (ed). Nutritional Toxicology Vol III, New York, Academic Press, 1989.

Macdonald I (ed). Monitoring Dietary Intakes. ILSI Monograph Berlin, Springer-Verlag, 1991.

INDEX